The Complete Book of

Yoga

and Meditation for

Pregnancy

The Complete Book of

Yoga
and
Meditation
for
Pregnancy

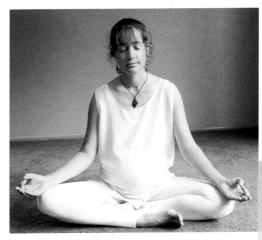

MILNER

Theresa Jamieson

First published in 2000 by

Sally Milner Publishing Pty Ltd

PO Box 2104

Bowral NSW 2576

AUSTRALIA

© Theresa Jamieson 2000

Reprinted 2000

Design Ken Gilroy

Photography Theresa Jamieson

Editing Lyneve Rappell

Artwork Beth Nelson

Index Deirdre Ward

Printed in Hong Kong

National Library of Australia Cataloguing-in-Publication data:

Jamieson, Theresa.

Yoga and meditation for pregnancy.

ISBN 1 86351 249 7

1. Exercise for pregnant women. 2. Meditation. 3. Yoga.

1. Title. (Series: Milner health series).

746.443

Disclaimer

The information in this instruction book is presented in good faith.

However, no warranty is given, nor results guaranteed,

nor is freedom from any patent to be inferred.

Since we have no control over the information contained

in this book, the publisher and the author disclaim liability

for untoward results.

DEDICATION

My book is about women's unique journey into motherhood, and honouring themselves during these brief and precious moments through the practice of yoga. It is also about the wonder of being a woman, the miracle of life itself and of women nurturing their inherent feminine wisdom, that is in each and every woman during pregnancy and birth.

They bring to form the celebration of life.

I dedicate my book to all women during their childbearing years and to their babes *in utero*.

Foreword

As a young inexperienced doctor, I first trained in a large city obstetric hospital. Even then, I was amazed at the high level of 'problem pregnancies' and intervention in labour.

When I left the city to work in the country, it became obvious that the management of pregnancies and labour was much different, with intervention less necessary. It was a lesson in how different the process of pregnancy and labour can be when the woman was relaxed and surrounded by 'at ease' staff and supportive family and friends.

After thirty years of being in general practice, I've found that the whole concept of preparation and labour has changed. It includes many more disciplines of care, and other skills and resources.

Yoga is one of the new disciplines that can enhance skills for the preparation of childbirth. It also encourages the development of skills that will be useful in parenting, and for immediate as well as subsequent personal, physical, emotional and spiritual aspects of life.

It has been obvious to me that women practising yoga for the childbirth preparation carry a new, and different dimension into this role, and their lives in general.

Theresa's book reflects this changed approach, and celebrates her own life and broad experience. Her extensive practice and teaching of yoga, in particular regard to pregnancy, childbirth and parenthood is apparent.

She expresses this experience readily to her readers, while her passion for the subject and her universal knowledge in what she writes about, produces a uniquely helpful reference and training manual for any woman about to prepare for pregnancy.

All women, and their support team, would do well to read and practise the guidance illustrated in this lifetime work.

Dr Robert Tiller
M.B.ChB. DipObs. DCommH.

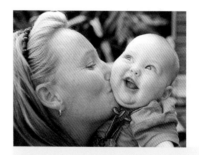

Contents

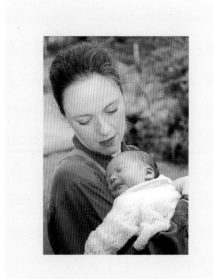

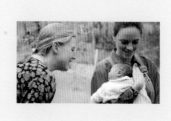

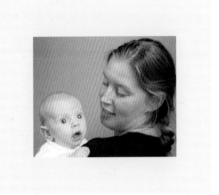

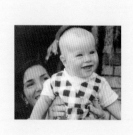

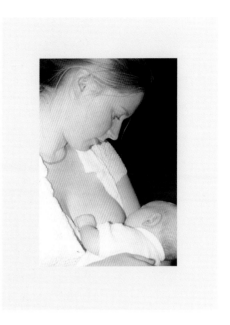

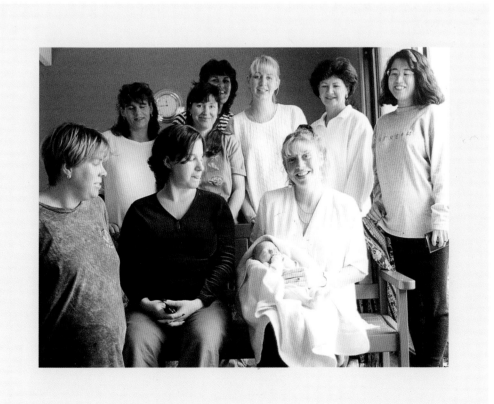

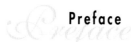

Preface

O ne of the most incredible rewards gained from practising the yoga *asanas* is to experience each movement as one of grace – where you come to recognise and perceive the subtle energies moving through you, at all times. When a posture is held, always be conscious of your breathing, how your body feels and where your thoughts are so the posture is always safe, centring and quite beautiful to do. By practising yoga in this way – with complete body, breath and mind awareness – you are fully conscious of the moment and are therefore in the process of observing the uniqueness and wonder of your whole body, mind and spirit.

Although pregnancy is a very brief moment in a lifetime, it is a precious opportunity to honour yourself as a woman, to acknowledge your actual pregnancy and your child *in utero*, while preparing for the ultimate joy of becoming a mother.

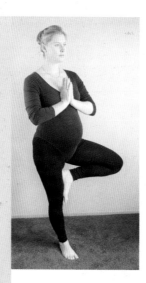

14

The complete book of
yoga and meditation
for pregnancy

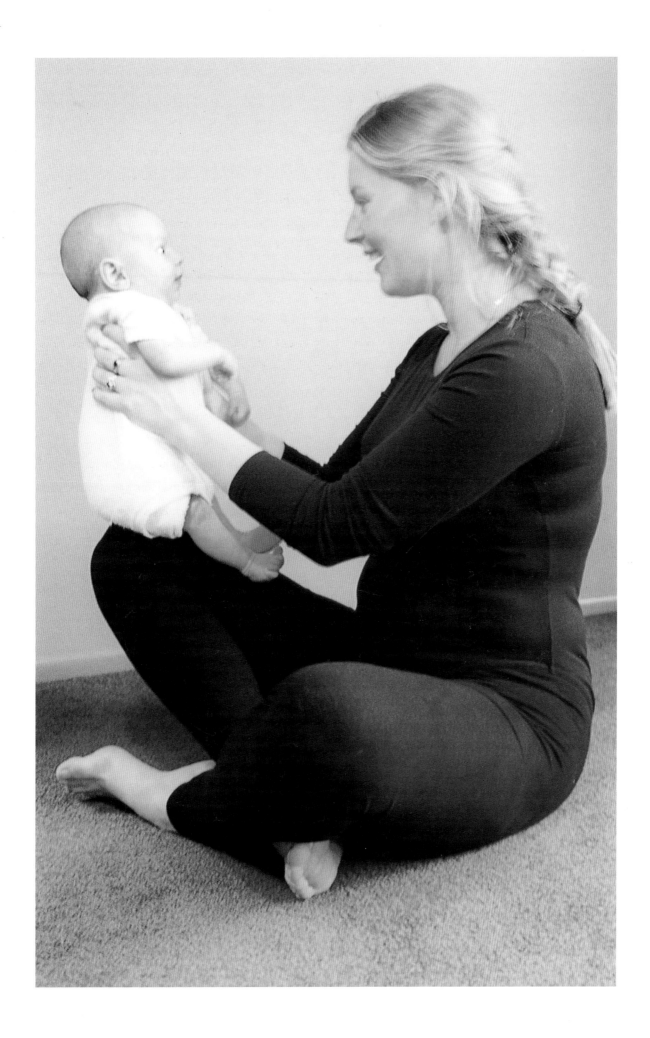

Acknowledgements

Acknowledgements

I would firstly like to thank my family, especially my husband Jeff and my children Ezra and Reuben, for being so patient with the completion of this book. Many times I would descend from the 'tower' to announce that it really is finished, only to spend many more weeks and even months on getting it right. My parents have also been encouraging and supportive all along, trusting the process much more than I was, and I thank them for that.

To Libby and Ian my publishers, for understanding my dream and bringing it to form and many thanks for encouraging 'my voice' to come forth in a safe and supportive environment. They enabled me to be courageous and forthright in an unfamiliar and new world. Thank you to Lyneve, whose job of editing my book has given it a readable and very easy format to work with.

I would like to thank Angela Chadwick from the college in Auckland for agreeing to my thesis topic and planting the initial seed for the completed book. To Dr John Barrett in Auckland who through his confidence in me and his referrals, created my first yoga classes for pregnant women. Without his encouragement and assistance I might have taken longer to realise where my path lay.

To Shantimurti in New Zealand for his brilliant and thorough teachings and to Bhaktimurti here on the Gold Coast, whose extraordinary insight and vast knowledge taught me so much more about yoga and meditation.

To my long suffering friends especially Robbie, Maree, Suzanne, Sandra, Susan, Trish, Christine, Joni, Jeanette, Debbie, Stewart and Fabian – to mention only a few for listening so patiently and consistently as I moved from one phase of the journey to another. A special thanks to my long time friend Yvonne (Quazz) for introducing me to yoga so many years ago, and Rosemary Moor my astrologer, who on numerous occasions helped ease my angst about the project, giving me the heavenly OK about completing the work. And to Chris and John O'Leary who are definitely a gift from the gods, for always, always being there for me with less than a moment's notice.

To Lorraine Woods at Pindara Private Hospital, a dear friend, who had enough faith in my yoga classes to go against tradition and include them into the antenatal program at the hospital, a decision that has provided young pregnant women with the opportunity to choose yoga as a valuable option if they so decided.

Thank you to my friend Paul who was always encouraging, but especially for being so challenging in regard to my fears and the many doubts I had along the way. Through this friendship I was fortunate enough to be introduced to the Venerable Khempo Migmar Tsering, who in such a brief space of time inspired my life and put my lack of self confidence in the project into perspective. Sadly he is no longer with us, but through his profound teachings and clear counsel he showed me the clarity I so needed to turn it all around and complete the book, thereby enabling me to reach many more

16

The complete book of
yoga and meditation
for pregnancy

pregnant women and ultimately help the refugee children of Tibet.

To Lynette Forgan-Gibbons for reading the text in the final moments. To my very talented friend Beth for the beautiful water colour art work of the herbs, and to Wendy for the arduous job of pulling it all together and giving it form to present to the publishers. Without her help the task would have been far more daunting than it was.

To the solicitors Price and Roobottom and to my lawyer Elizabeth Gore-Jones, for so generously donating their services for the legal work. As all the proceeds are being donated to the Tibetan Children's Village in India, I feel their contribution should be applauded as an honourable and unique thing to do. I am very blessed to have them working for me and for the realisation of my dream.

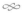

Finally, I would like to thank all the women who came to my home for the photographs, always so late in their pregnancies and often in hot and uncomfortable weather. A special thanks to Tori who the majority of photographs are taken of, I really appreciate the time and effort you gave during your pregnancy and after the birth as well. To the 11 women who took their time so soon after the birth to write their personal accounts of their birthing experience, many thanks for bringing your wonderful stories to the world. Thank you also to Eva for taking the time to drive the distance from your hinterland home on two occasions, for the cover photo. I feel your beauty, grace and absolute contentment shines through as you reflect on your baby in

the womb. Your photo has captured the true essence of what the book is ultimately all about.

And finally to all the women I have met over the years of teaching, who by attending my classes continuously have shown me what really works best and feels right for the pregnant woman – you really have been my greatest teachers.

The photographs

Most of the photos in this book are of Tori but I have also photographed a number of other women doing the postures and exercises with ease and grace. I hope this will encourage more women to try practising yoga no matter what their age, degree of flexibility, stage of pregnancy or past experience with yoga.

When the photographs were taken, Tori was 39 weeks; Sandra was 39.5 weeks; Lindsay was 12 days over her due date; Darani, Clare, Karon, Narelle, Eva and Veronica were 38 weeks and Janelle was 33 weeks pregnant with twins.

The watercolours

The beautiful watercolours were painted by my dear friend, Beth Nelson, who has exhibited and sold many fine pieces of art in Australia and New Zealand. Her expression of the herbs is quite exquisite and a wonderful contribution to the book. The herbs she has painted are specifically relevant to pregnant women both during pregnancy and after birth. Most importantly, they are also safe to use.

Introduction

The thoughts and feelings expressed in this book have come from my own experiences during pregnancy and the privileged time I have had with many pregnant women over years of teaching.

This book comes from an intense desire to share the wonders of yoga for pregnancy with all women, no matter how young or old they are or how fit or unfit they might be. Practising yoga during pregnancy gives women the opportunity to take time out to honour this special time in their lives and to appreciate the gift of the life inside them.

Women have a variety of individual needs during pregnancy so I am not able to guarantee that practising yoga will be the wonderful experience it has been for most of the women I have met. However, if a little time is given to practising and understanding the different techniques – even if only to observe the breath moving in and out of your body – I feel sure that some aspect of yoga will make a favourable contribution to your pregnancy, labour, birth and recovery.

After I have practiced yoga, I always notice a feeling of lightness and freedom of movement. With ongoing practise, we begin to discover a peaceful, gentle place at the very centre of our being. It is like coming home to ourselves.

A balanced program

To gain the greatest rewards from yoga, I feel all aspects of this ancient art should be practised including; *asana*, *pranayama*, some form of meditation, and deep relaxation. I also feel that women of all ages – but particularly around childbirth – should practise Pelvic Floor exercises every day.

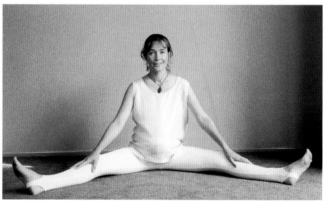

Asana

Primarily, the asanas will tone, strengthen and stretch your whole body while also helping to release any tightness, tension or stiffness from your muscles. They will help to develop greater flexibility and suppleness. Stretch and strength are equalised and balanced on both sides of your body. The health of the nervous system is improved and harmonised, while the health of the endocrine glands, the function of the digestive system and the musculoskeletal systems are also dramatically improved. Circulation is increased to all areas of the body and an enriched blood supply combined with greater oxygen utilisation has an overall nourishing effect. The end result is a much improved sense of wellbeing and far less fatigue. However, of most significance for the purposes of this

18

The complete book of
yoga and meditation
for pregnancy

book are the benefits that yoga has for the female reproductive system, as it provides a gentle, safe and supportive health care program for both mother and baby during pregnancy and after birth.

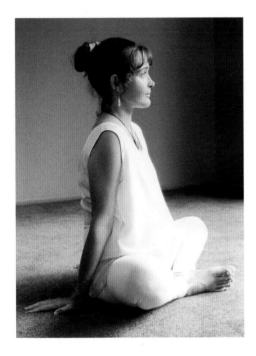

Pranayama

While the *asana*s are obviously very significant in themselves, pranayama is also invaluable. When we breathe more efficiently, oxygen utilisation and uptake are improved. This life giving oxygen reaches every cell so that your whole body is positively affected and recharged with energy. In yoga, this vital energy is known as prana or the life force. In addition, the habit of correct breathing encourages deeper relaxation in your body, and your mind becomes calmer and more stable.

Meditation & Relaxation

Yoga is also an invaluable tool for mental and emotional wellbeing. Alongside *asana* and *pranayama*,

meditation *(dhyana)* and deep relaxation *(yoga nidra)* are able to help in turning off your mind. They give us time out from our busy lives and space to stand apart from the dramas of our lives. They allow us a little peace within the course of each day. The time spent in meditation or deep relaxation need only be 10 or 15 minutes each day, but the result of this process is true rest and rejuvenation at all levels. These practices are important in relieving stress and tension. In conjunction with other therapies, many mental or emotional problems can be better managed with the assistance of these gentle yoga practices.

Getting started

In the section Antenatal Programs you will find the chapters 'Six Half-hour Programs' and 'Salute to the Sun, Modified'. You may like to begin with some of the half-hour programs until you become familiar with the book and able to select the exercises which suit you best. As you become comfortable with practising yoga regularly you may like to try the modified version of the Salute to the Sun.

You might notice a tightness in your muscles when you first start practising yoga, especially if you have not been doing some other form of stretching exercises. Don't be dismayed if this happens. It usually disappears after a few classes. Other forms of exercise tend to tighten the muscles rather than give them flexibility so care needs to be taken when you first commence yoga, even if you are a very fit person.

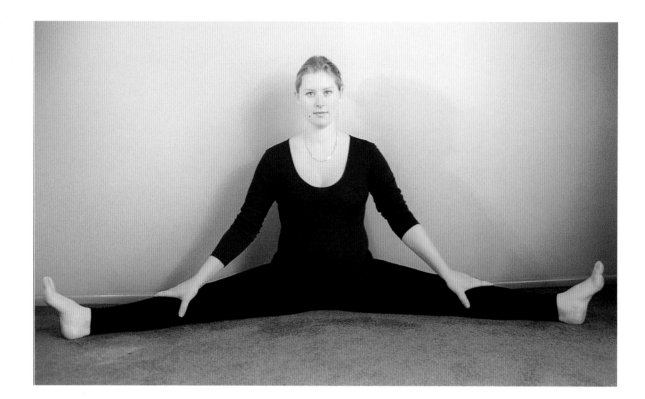

Generally, yoga is practised when the bowels and bladder are empty, and at least three hours after a meal. If you have a problem with hypoglycemia or diabetes, eat a small amount before practising the postures and, if need be, snack on dry biscuits during the class.

When you are doing the exercises on the floor, use a thin rubber floor mat which is the length of your body. Wear loose, comfortable clothing that does not constrict your chest or waist. Practise yoga in a room that is free of draughts or direct sunlight, and move any furniture that may hinder your movements.

In the hotter weather, drink plenty of water to prevent dehydration. During the cooler months, cover your body with a blanket when you are in the resting positions. Wear socks for the relaxation and meditation practices because your body temperature will drop when you relax.

The number nine

I have used the number nine throughout this book because it represents the nine months of pregnancy. I have also used it as a general guide to the number of breaths a posture can be held for and as a reference in the breathing exercises and meditation.

The number nine is a special number. It is the number of completion and eternity. The Chinese favoured nine, believing it to be auspicious. They incorporated it into their society with nine social laws and nine classes of officials. It is also three times three.

Number three appears as a symbol of the trinity in a number of religions. In Christianity there is the father, the son and the holy ghost. In Hinduism there is Shiva, Vishnu and Brahma. Three is especially important because it underlies all aspects of creation: body, mind and spirit; birth, life and death; and past, present and future; and, of course, three trimesters of pregnancy.

20

The complete book of
yoga and meditation
for pregnancy

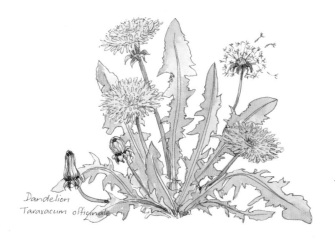

Dandelion
Taraxacum officinale

What is Yoga?

To understand what yoga is, it is best to start with the meaning of the word. The word yoga comes from the Sanskrit word *yuj* which means to join, to unify, a coming together or a yoke. The practice of yoga is a union of the whole person – the soul, the mind, the emotions and the physical body. It is a coming together of our human selves with the more divine aspects of our being – that is, our higher consciousness, our divinity, or the way we interpret God in our lives. It is both spiritual and physical in nature. When yoga is practised regularly, we develop a deeper and more profound understanding of the spiritual aspects of our nature while our physical selves become more balanced and harmonious.

Archeological evidence suggests that yoga has been around for more than 10,000 years. Statues depicting yoga postures and meditation positions from that time have been discovered in the Indus Valley which is in Pakistan.

The first books on yoga were written around that time and are known as the *Vedas*. They are considered to be the most sacred books of Hindu literature. Included in the *Vedas* are the *Upanishads* which are the philosophical part of the *Vedas*.

The first systemic writing on yoga was put together by the sage, Patanjali. His text is called the *Yoga Sutra* and is still closely followed today. Patanjali's work is often referred to (Iyengar 1966, p. 3) as the Eight Fold Path consisting of:

1. Yama - self restraint
2. Niyama - self observation
3. Asana - physical postures
4. Pranayama - breathing exercises
5. Pratyahara - becoming less associated with the outside world, withdrawal of the consciousness from the external environment
6. Dharana - concentration
7. Dhyana - meditation
8. Samadi - ultimate awareness of pure consciousness

These eight aspects of yoga provide an excellent guideline for any yoga practitioner to follow, while being also one of the paths ascribed to for a better understanding of the self and ultimately to self realisation.

Yoga is the control of the waves of the mind. Normally the self is identified with these waves, but it is possible to free it so that it rests on its own.

(Patanjali in Hutchinson 1974)

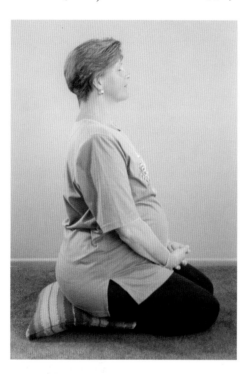

There are many forms of yoga but it is the practice of Hatha Yoga which is detailed in this book. It is interesting to realise that even when Hatha Yoga is taken up purely as a form of physical exercise where the body becomes more agile, supple and relaxed, that the inner calmness experienced seems to naturally overflow to the mental, emotional and spiritual aspects of the personality, thereby positively effecting the whole person.

I will be dealing primarily with: the physical exercises *(asanas)*; the breathing exercises *(pranayama)*, the gestures *(mudras)*; meditation *(dhyana)*; and deep relaxation *(yoga nidra)*. I feel it

is important to mention here that in its truest form, Hatha Yoga did not consist of these practices. It was a series of advanced cleansing techniques that are still practised today by very experienced yogis. However, Hatha Yoga is the term most commonly used to describe the system that is taught today.

One traditional yogic teaching is called Tantra Yoga, which involves the *chakra* system. There are seven major *chakras*, or energy centres, located within the spiritual body and these are situated along the inside of the spinal column from the base of the spine to the top of the head. The *chakras* are connected to each other by psychic channels called *nadis*. On a physical level, *nadis* are comparable to the network of nerves that connect to the central nervous system. Energy, or *prana*, flows throughout the psychic body along these *nadis*, and in a similar but more physical sense, the nerves send energy via messages and nerve impulses to the physical body.

In the middle of the physical body we have the spinal column and corresponding to this the most important *nadi* is found, known as *sushumna nadi*.

There are apparently 72,000 *nadis* in the body, and the main ones cross each other at the *chakra* points on the inside of the spinal column. In yogic teachings, these *nadis* are the pathways for *prana* to flow to our whole being. In a similar way the nervous system in our physical bodies sends messages throughout the whole body via the nerves, while in Chinese tradition the meridians are pathways where *chi* or energy is carried within the person.

When any of these systems are balanced, the person will feel well and move through life easily and in peace, but where there is an imbalance the

22

The complete book of
yoga and meditation
for pregnancy

person might begin to feel unwell and physical problems will emerge. This is also true in regard to the health of the emotions, which can be thrown out of balance because of the many stresses that are part of our daily lives. From a Western point of view, there are various therapies and medicines for maintaining health in the nervous system. In Chinese philosophy, acupuncture and herbal remedies are used for recreating health.

When the yoga postures are practised, even in their simplest forms, we are not only working on the physical body but are also stimulating and balancing our *chakra* system. Every posture we do affects both our physical and psychic bodies. In this way, harmony is established in the body, mind and spirit.

When applying the ancient skills and teachings of yoga through ongoing practice, we have the opportunity to form a 'communion' with ourselves or to create a union with our entire nature, which allows us to then embrace what yoga means in its simplest yet truest form. This enables us to come together more as an individual, to merge our outer and inner selves more completely and to discover a peaceful, gentle place at the very centre of our beings.

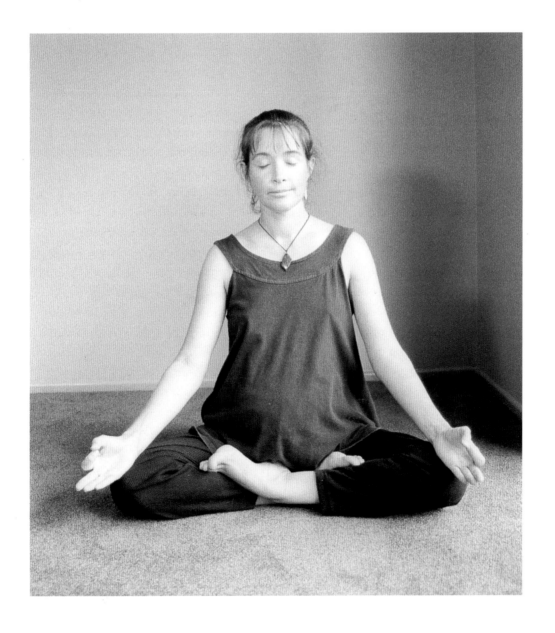

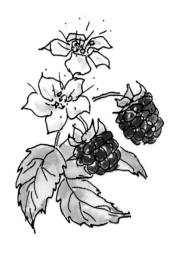

Yoga for Pregnancy

Is it safe?

Yoga during pregnancy provides a gentle, safe and supportive health care program for both mother and baby. Before you begin the exercises in this book or yoga classes, however, always discuss your intentions with your doctor or midwife to ensure there is no reason why yoga would not be suitable and to give you a feeling of confidence before commencing.

If you have had a miscarriage in the past, if you have a history of threatened miscarriages or if you have any concerns about pregnancy, it would be wise to begin the physical exercises *(asanas)* after the fourth month of pregnancy. However, you can commence the breathing exercises *(pranayama)*, meditation and relaxation practices as soon as possible after conception. If you have a disability or a delicate health condition, you should consult a skilled yoga teacher to modify the practices to suit your needs.

The physical exercises I have recommended are quite specific for pregnant women. They can assist, throughout the pregnancy, by increasing physical tone and strength. They are designed to work specifically on the parts of your body most involved in pregnancy, to allow optimum organ function and health. They are also of value after the birth in ensuring a faster return to your pre-pregnancy level of fitness.

Care needs to be taken at all times not to overdo the practices but, at the same time, not to practise so infrequently as to feel no benefit at all. Discontinue a posture if you feel faint, light headed, dizzy or nauseous. Do not practise the physical exercises if you are tired but instead practise meditation, relaxation or breathing. This will help to restore your energies rather than deplete them.

24

The complete book of
yoga and meditation
for pregnancy

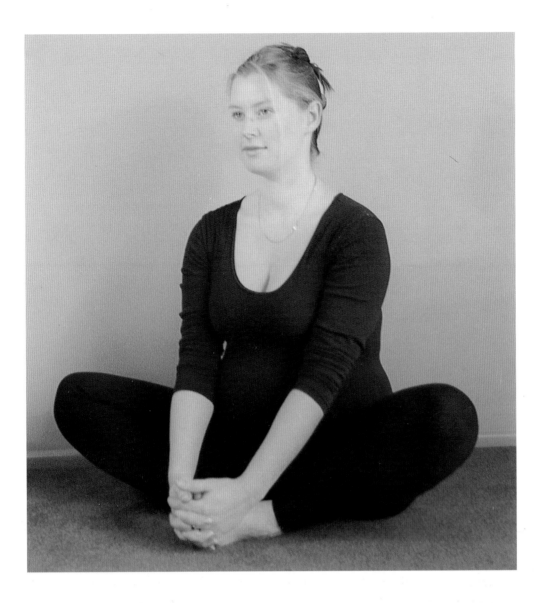

When should I start yoga?

It is not necessary to have practised yoga before conception. Many women only find out about yoga when they are well into their pregnancies and don't start classes until the last few weeks. Although this is not a perfect situation, a number of women have told me how much benefit they received during labour even after attending only one or two classes. The skills learnt during that time might be the very ones needed during labour. It is definitely a case of 'better late than never'. Ideally, however, it is more rewarding to begin classes before conception or as soon after as possible.

How often do I need to practise?

Although yoga is a system of many different and specific practices, it is also quite a personal study. You need to be aware of what feels right for you as you progress with your pregnancy. You will know, better than anybody else, how you are feeling from day to day and it is important to discontinue a particular practice if you feel it is no longer suitable for you. Listen to your own intuition about how much and how often to practise. Every woman will approach pregnancy in a different way and the practices and guidelines are there for you to follow at your own pace to ensure you have a happy and healthy pregnancy.

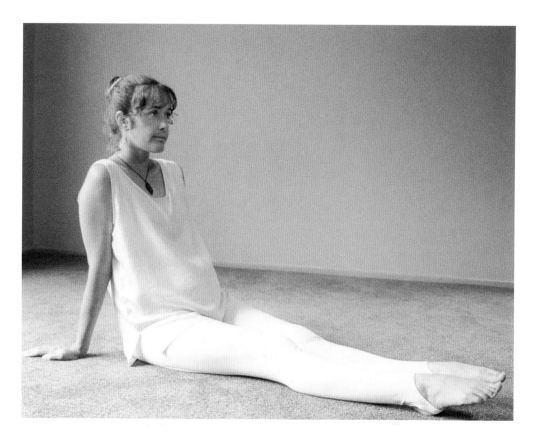

Ankle exercises

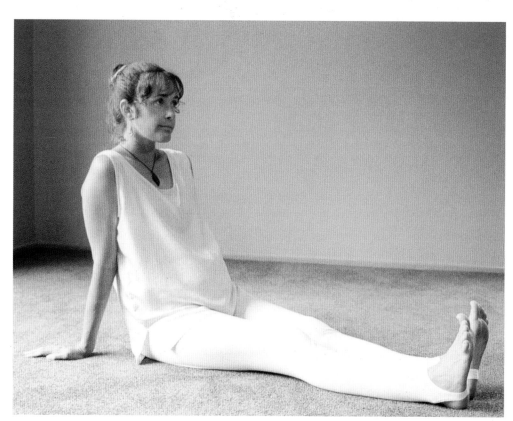

The complete book of
yoga and meditation
for pregnancy

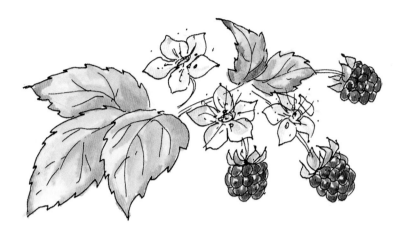

ASANA
Warming Up

You are where your attention takes you. In fact, you are your attention. If your attention is fragmented, you are fragmented. When your attention is in the past, you are in the past. When your attention is in the present moment, you are in the presence of God and God is present in you.

(Chopra 1993, p. 61)

These warming up exercises and gentle yoga postures are an excellent way to tone and loosen your body before practising the other postures, or *asanas*. They can also be practised on their own and they are especially useful if you are feeling a little weaker than usual or if your doctor has suggested a light yoga program.

I suggest before commencing that you spend a little time in one of the relaxation postures with your awareness on breathing deeply and quietly. This will help relax your body, quieten your mind and focus your thoughts in the present moment.

1. Ankle exercises

These simple movements will help relieve fluid retention in your ankles and feet, especially in the later weeks of pregnancy.

1. Sit on the floor with your back straight and your legs in front of you. Lean against a wall if necessary or use cushions behind your back for extra comfort.

2. Point your toes down slowly. Next, flex your feet up so that you can feel a deep stretch through the tops of your feet and in your calf muscles. Repeat this exercise up to nine times.

3. Spread your toes wide apart and then squeeze them tightly together. Do this up to nine times.

4. Slowly rotate your ankles clockwise five times and then anticlockwise five times. Make the circles large and slow to work deeply into your feet and ankles. This exercise will also help to reduce swelling and it is a good preparation for the Lotus and Half Lotus postures.

2. Hand and Finger exercises

These exercises help maintain flexibility in your wrists, hands and fingers, and improve circulation in your lower arms. They are especially useful if your hands are inclined to swell in hot weather. They can be practised either sitting in a traditional posture, in a chair with your back straight, or standing with your feet a little apart.

1. Stretch your arms out in front of you at shoulder height. Spread your fingers wide apart. Squeeze your hands into tight fists. Repeat this up to nine times. Lightly shake your hands when you have completed the exercise.

3. Shoulder exercises
(skandhachakra)

This group of exercises helps free tension from your shoulders. They assist in opening up your chest for more efficient breathing and they also help prevent incorrect posture and round shoulders.

1. Stand with your feet slightly apart and your body relaxed. Place your fingertips on your shoulders.

2. Make slow, large circles with your elbows so that your shoulders are rotating deeply in their sockets. Repeat this nine times forwards and then nine times backwards. When your elbows are

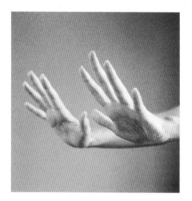 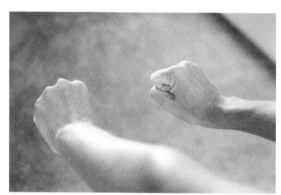 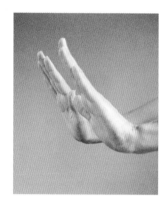

2. Clench your fists and very slowly rotate them clockwise nine times and then anticlockwise nine times. As you do this, be aware of the stretch throughout your wrists and arms.

3. Stretch your arms out in front of you at shoulder height with your palms facing down. Flex your hands upwards so that the palms of your hands are facing away from you and your fingers are pointing up. Reverse the movement and point your fingers down towards the floor. Repeat this five times, then lightly shake your hands.

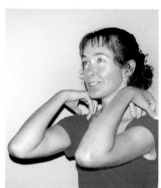 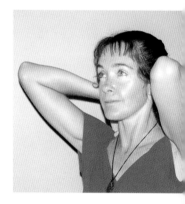

forward, the stretch will be felt across your upper back and shoulders helping to relieve any tension in these parts of your body. As your elbows are back, the stretch is felt in your chest. Although this is a simple exercise, the way your back and shoulders will feel afterwards is evidence enough of its benefits.

28

The complete book of
yoga and meditation
for pregnancy

Lightly shake your arms and loosen your shoulders after the exercise is completed.

4. Head and Neck exercises
(gardhanasana)

These exercises reduce tension in your neck and shoulders. Your neck plays a vital role in overall health because nerves from various parts of your body pass through your neck to your brain. If you are suffering from headaches and neck tension, regular practice of these exercises will provide you with welcome relief. At the very least, it should prevent the problem becoming worse.

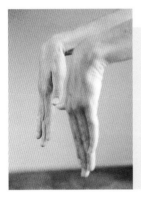

Caution: I do not recommend a full head rotation for anyone. This is especially relevant if you have a weak or injured neck.

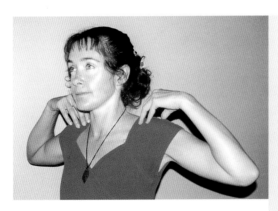

These three exercises are best done slowly, with your upper body relaxed and your back straight. They can be done from a standing position, sitting in a chair or sitting on the floor.

1. Lower your head towards your right shoulder, being careful not to lift your shoulder or become tense. Remember to keep the muscles in your neck and shoulders relaxed. Do not force your head over towards your shoulder in any way and only go as far as is comfortable. Hold this position for four or five breaths and then repeat it to the left. This whole exercise can be repeated as many times as desired. The weight of your head will gently stretch the muscles at the side of your neck so there is no need to force the position. It is worth doing this exercise in front of a mirror to make sure your body is not leaning as you move your head.

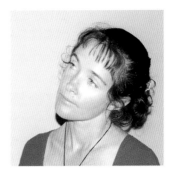

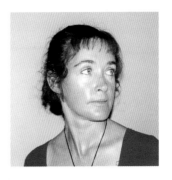

2. Turn your head as far to the right as possible, holding it for a short time before turning it to the left. Repeat this five times each side, keeping your neck and shoulders relaxed.

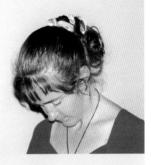

3. Drop your head down so that your chin is close to your chest. Be aware of feeling a deep stretch through the muscles of your upper back, shoulders and the central muscles of your neck. Your head can also be taken back but I do not recommend this if you have had a neck injury. If you are able to take your head back comfortably, slowly open and close your mouth so as to stretch the muscles of your throat. Again, the weight of your head will automatically cause your neck muscles to be stretched.

5. Eye exercises
(neytrasana)

Our eyes are so important in everyday life that it seems only natural we should exercise our eyes as we exercise other parts of our body. Many eye specialist now recommend similar eye exercises as part of their health care program. These exercises are easy to do and take only a short time. They help relieve eye strain, improve vision and act as a safeguard against eye problems in the future.

These exercises can be practised from any comfortable seated position with your back straight and relaxed. If you wear contact lenses or glasses you might elect to remove them before you start, but this is not necessary. Blink your eyes whenever you need to and if you feel a little light headed when practising the exercises, close your eyes until the sensation has passed and before proceeding on with the other exercises.

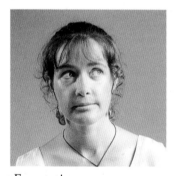

Eye rotations

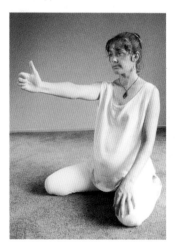

Eye rotations

Eye rotations
Roll your eyes in circles by slowly rotating them five times to the right and then five times to the left. Rest with your eyes closed and repeat once more if desired.

Eyes to the right and to the left
1. Stretch your right arm out in front of you, raising it to eye height. Gaze at your right thumb. Slowly move your arm as far to the right as you are able to without straining your eyes or moving your head. Follow your thumb as you return your arm to the centre

front and repeat the movement twice more. Lower your arm and rest with your eyes closed.

2. Repeat the same movements with your left arm raised. Remember it is important not to turn your head or strain your eyes in this exercise. Again, rest with your eyes closed when you have finished.

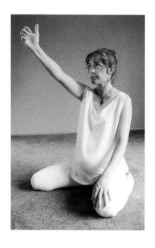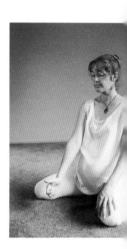

Eyes up and down
1. Stretch your right arm out in front of you at eye height. Gaze at your thumb. Slowly raise your arm up in front of you as high as possible, without tilting your head back or straining your eyes.

2. Slowly lower your arm, continuing to watch your thumb, towards the floor. Again, do not move your head or strain your eyes. Repeat this movement (of lifting and lowering your arm) three times.

3. When finished, rest with your eyes closed.

Slow circles
1. Begin with your right arm raised to eye height. Gaze at your right thumb. To complete a slow half circle, move your right arm up as high as possible and then make a wide half circle to the right, finishing at the bottom centre front.

2. From the centre front your left arm completes the circle, starting from the bottom left then out to the left as wide as possible, to the centre top.

3. Lower your left arm and rest before repeating the circle in the opposite direction, reversing all the movements. When complete, rest with your eyes closed. Repeat three times.

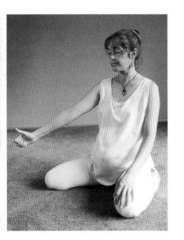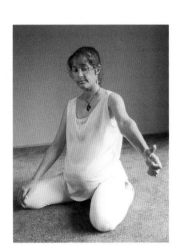

Looking at a close and distant object

1. Gaze at the tip of your nose, without straining. Then rest with your eyes closed. Repeat this up to nine times.

2. Focus your vision on an object in the distance and hold your gaze for two or three minutes.

3. Alternate from a close object to a distant object. Read a book at a normal distance from your face and then gradually move the book away to be further away from your normal viewing range. This will help to improve your long sight as well as your closer, more detailed vision.

4. Hold your arm at eye height, gazing at your thumb. Slowly move your thumb in towards your face to touch your nose, before moving it away from you. Repeat this three times.

Palming

Traditionally, hands have been associated with healing and comfort. This exercise has a very soothing effect and is recommended as a special procedure to do at the end of the eye exercises.

1. Simply rub the palms of your hands together vigorously until they feel warm. Hold your palms over your eyes in the shape of a shallow cup. Keep them in that position until you notice the warmth has cooled from your hands and then repeat this three times, once with your eyes closed, once with them open and once while blinking your eyes rapidly. This whole exercise can be repeated whenever you have tired or irritated eyes, especially from long hours of reading or working on a computer.

Full moon gazing

On a clear, full-moon night, look directly at the moon. The light from the sun is reflected by the surface of the moon so it isn't harmful to your eyes. Apart from being a very pleasant thing to do, it also revitalises your eyes by stimulating the optic nerve.

Gazing at the rising and setting sun

It is important to only look at the rising sun for the first seven or eight minutes. To look for longer can damage your eyes. Obviously, you will need to be in a place where you are actually able to see these first few minutes of sunrise. The last nine or ten minutes of the setting sun is also beneficial for your

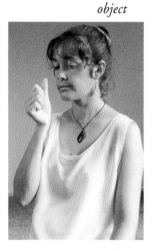

Looking at a close object

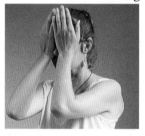

Palming

eyes, and again you need to be in a place where this is possible. If you are fortunate enough to see either the sunrise or the sunset it is a beautiful and calming for both your body and your mind.

There are many places in the world where it is possible to see the first moments of the sun touching the earth, as well as the last moments before it lights the other side of the earth. On the Indonesian island of Bali it is possible to see both the sunrise and sunset from different sides of the island.

On a personal note, I remember a remarkable evening on the west coast of India, where the golden sun was setting into the Arabian Sea before me, and at the same moment a huge full moon was rising, between the coconut palms, behind me. It was extraordinary, because both were at the same height and both were perfectly round and brilliant. It was a rare moment when *Hamstring* day and night were truly held in the *stretches* balance.

muscles. These gentle exercises are an ideal way to loosen the hamstrings but it is important not to lift your leg any higher than is comfortable for you. It is better to hold your leg straight, but a little lower, than to lean back or bend your leg in an effort to raise it higher. With regular practice your hamstrings and leg muscles will become more flexible. These stretches can also improve circulation to your legs.

1. Sit on the floor with your back straight and your legs in front of you. If you find it difficult to sit unsupported with your back straight, resting against a wall will make it easier.

2. Bend your right leg and place your hands under your knee, keeping your left leg straight on the floor. Keep your back straight for the whole practice.

3. Breathe in and straighten your right leg, holding it as high as possible without bending your knee.

4. Breathe out as you lower your leg to the floor. Repeat the exercise,

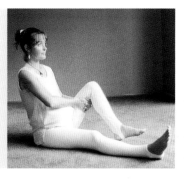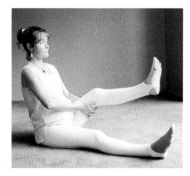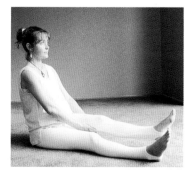

Trataka, the Candle Meditation is another excellent exercises for your eyes and can be practiced in conjunction with the eye exercises.

6. Hamstring Stretches
(janu naman)

Hamstring tendons and thigh muscles are often tight to the point where people cringe at the thought of doing the postures that work these

with the same leg, five times or more.

5. Repeat this exercise with your left leg.

7. Hip Rotations
(shoni chakra)

The Hip Rotations are an important exercise for pregnancy and can be used as a preparation for postures that involve the hips, such as the Butterfly, Squatting, the Wide-A Leg

32

The complete book of
yoga and meditation
for pregnancy
∞

Stretches and the Crescent Moon. The exercise will tone and open your pelvic area, while giving increased flexibility and freedom of movement to your hips. It might feel quite awkward to begin with but if you concentrate on making large circles with your knee, rather than with your hip, you will find it less difficult. Always approach it slowly, making big circles in both directions.

1. Sit on the floor with your spine straight and your legs in front of you.

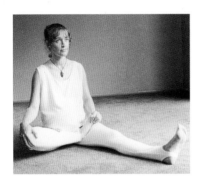

2. Bend your right leg. Hold onto your right foot with you left hand and your right knee with your right hand.

3. Make slow circles with the right knee so as to rotate your whole hip. Repeat this five times in a clockwise direction and five times in an anticlockwise direction. Shake you leg lightly when you have completed the exercise.

4. Repeat the exercise rotating your left hip.

8. The Half Butterfly

The Half Butterfly posture is an excellent way to prepare for the Butterfly and other postures where flexibility is required in your hip and inner thigh areas.

1. Sit on the floor with your back straight and relaxed. Your left leg is straight and your right knee is bent. Rest your right foot on top of your left

thigh, or if this is not comfortable, place the sole of your right foot beside your left thigh. Your ankle needs to be quite supple before your foot can comfortably be placed on top of your thigh, but with regular practice of the exercises for your feet and the hip rotations, greater flexibility will be achieved over time.

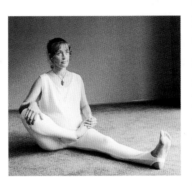

2. Hold onto your foot and your knee and bounce your right leg freely up and down without straining. Practise this movement nine times or more before changing legs and repeating it with your left leg. Some women are naturally very flexible in the hip and inner thigh areas and will find these practices much easier than other women. Don't worry if your knee doesn't reach the floor when you first begin. With time, you will become more open and supple.

9. The Butterfly
(baddhakonasana)

The Butterfly is probably one of the most important seated positions to consider as an antenatal exercise. It is recommended in most yoga books and exercise classes as an ideal preparation for pregnancy. Your whole pelvic region, your inner thighs and your hips are 'opened' and toned, without any stress being applied to these parts of your body. The abductor muscles of your inner thigh are stretched and strengthened. The Butterfly improves circulation as well as kidney and bladder function. Your reproductive system is balanced, establishing excellent organ function and integrity. It has been found that women who sit in this posture regularly are more likely to have an easier delivery and recovery after the birth, as is also the case with the Squatting exercises.

It is very important not to force your knees towards the ground or strain yourself in any way. The movement of your knees should be gentle and relaxed. When you first practise the Butterfly, spend some time sitting with the soles of your feet together. If you discover you are tight in your inner thigh area, sit with your back against a wall for extra support and, if need be, sit on a small cushion. Cushions can be placed under your knees for support and as your flexibility increases these can be removed.

suppleness. You will also feel a much deeper stretch if you place your hands behind your buttocks, and actually move your buttocks in towards your feet, rather than your feet in towards your buttocks. For extra expansion and stretch, place your hands on your knees and very gently press on your knees to ease them towards the floor, remembering you are always the best judge of how deep the stretch needs to be and at no time feeling you have 'opened' too far.

To increase your flexibility, the Butterfly posture can be practised lying on your back, either on the floor or on a bed or with your buttocks, legs and feet against a wall. If you find this a

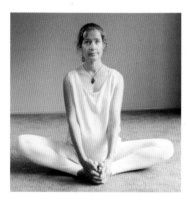
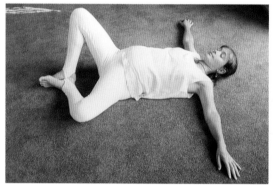
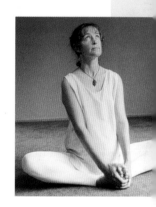

Variation (i)

1. Sit with your back straight and relaxed, the soles of your feet together and your hands holding onto your feet. If you feel the stretch is too strong, place a cushion under each knee for extra support.

2. With gentle movements, move your knees up and down like a butterfly's wings, remembering not to force your legs towards the floor. The object of this exercise, is to open and stretch your inner thigh and pelvic area without forcing your legs onto the floor. I have seen many women who are initially quite stiff when attempting this exercise, but with a little patience and regular practice they soon achieve more

comfortable position, it can be used for resting and relaxing. The effects of gravity are greater when lying on your back and your knees will naturally fall towards the floor. As there is virtually no pressure on your back in this lying down position, it is better for those who have a weak lower back or back pain during the last trimester. Cushions can be placed under your knees in the lying position, also.

Variation (ii)

1. From the Butterfly posture, breathe in as you stretch your knees towards the floor while lifting up your feet with your hands. Straighten your back and look upwards.

34

The complete book of
yoga and meditation
for pregnancy

2. Breathe out and bring your head towards your feet. Press your elbows lightly into your calf muscles as your knees are eased towards the floor. Keep your shoulders relaxed at all times.

3. Repeat these two movements up to nine times, breathing in and out rhythmically as you move from position 1 to position 2. When you inhale, try to straighten your back and stretch fully

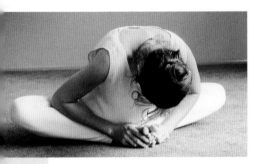

Left & above: The Butterfly (Var. ii)

throughout your spinal column, feeling the upward lift of your body, and the opposite sensation in your legs as you bend over and your knees are pressed to the floor.

10. The Thunderbolt
(vajrasana)

The Thunderbolt, or Diamond, posture is used as a seated position by many cultures. It is famous as the posture adopted by Japanese Buddhists for meditation and prayer. It is a very comfortable posture to use for resting and quietening your mind, for practising the breathing exercises *(pranayama)*, and during meditation.

If you find sitting in this posture uncomfortable, a small cushion can be placed between your calf muscles and the backs of your thighs to relieve any discomfort in your knees. A thin piece of foam padding can be placed under your feet until your ankles and feet become accustomed to having weight on them.

This posture helps improve circulation to your pelvis and other internal organs. Your pelvic floor muscles are also strengthened. It is probably one of the most beneficial positions to sit in after a meal because your spine is straight and the digestive processes can function more efficiency. This is very important during pregnancy, as many women suffer from indigestion. For those with peptic ulcers, hyperacidity, heartburn and bloating after eating, it is the preferred position to bring relief from those problems. Your ankles and the muscles of your feet are stretched and loosened, helping relieve arthritis in your hips and your knees.

When this position is first practised, remain in the position for a short time only so as to avoid unnecessary discomfort in your feet and ankles. If you have varicose veins do not remain in the position for extended periods.

1. Sit in a kneeling position with your knees together, your big toes touching and your heels apart. Your buttocks should rest on your feet or, if need be, on a cushion.

2. Make sure your back is relaxed and your spine is straight.

3. Place the palms of your hands face-down on top of your thighs. Bend your elbows slightly to prevent tension in your arms and shoulders.

11. The Frog (mandukasana) with arm exercises

The Frog is an excellent posture for pregnancy and for after the birth. It has all the benefits of the two previous postures as well as stretching deeply into your inner thigh muscles due to the wide position of your legs. It is very useful for relieving tension throughout your hips, pelvic floor and whole pelvic and abdominal region, being especially important to the health of the female reproductive system and bladder.

These arm exercises are one of the few where the muscles of your upper arms are toned, firmed and strengthened. However, if you find the Frog uncomfortable to hold, it is not necessary to do the arm exercises from that position. Any other seated position where your back is straight and relaxed would also be suitable.

1. Sit in the Thunderbolt posture and widen your knees as far as possible. Sit on your heels and have your big toes crossed or touching. A cushion can be placed under your buttocks for extra comfort. Feel your whole body relax.

2. Take your arms up above your head. Join your palms together and rest the heels of your hands on the crown of your head. Your shoulders stay down and relaxed throughout the exercise.

3. Breathe in as you raise and straighten your arms above your head, while pressing the palms of your hands together. If you push too hard you will cause strain and tension in your upper arms and shoulders.

4. Breathe out as the heels of your hands are lowered to the top of your head.

5. Repeat this as many times as you like, being aware of the strong sensations in your upper arms and chest. It is important not to repeat this so often that your arms ache or become fatigued, remembering it is quite a strenuous posture which requires strength in your upper arms and shoulders. I usually suggest repeating this five or six times and by then most people are feeling the effects of the exercise and are ready to lower their arms.

6. When you have completed the exercise, lower your arms and lightly shake your arms and hands. Stretch your legs out in front of you, shaking them lightly to restore the circulation and remove any stiffness from sitting in the Frog posture.

12. The Head of the Cow (gomukhasana)

The Head of the Cow is another ideal exercise for your arms and shoulders. It can be done from any seated position where your back is straight and relaxed. You might notice it much easier to do on one side than the other, but with regular practice both sides will eventually balance. *Gomukhasana*, when translated means one of two things. Go means cow and mukha is face, indicating the face of a cow, but a Gomukha is also a musical instrument that is broad at one end and narrow at the other, like a cow's face.

This posture works deeply into your shoulders, upper arms and neck muscles. It is useful for relieving tension in these areas, as well as being helpful for the relief of backache.

36

The complete book of
yoga and meditation
for pregnancy

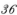

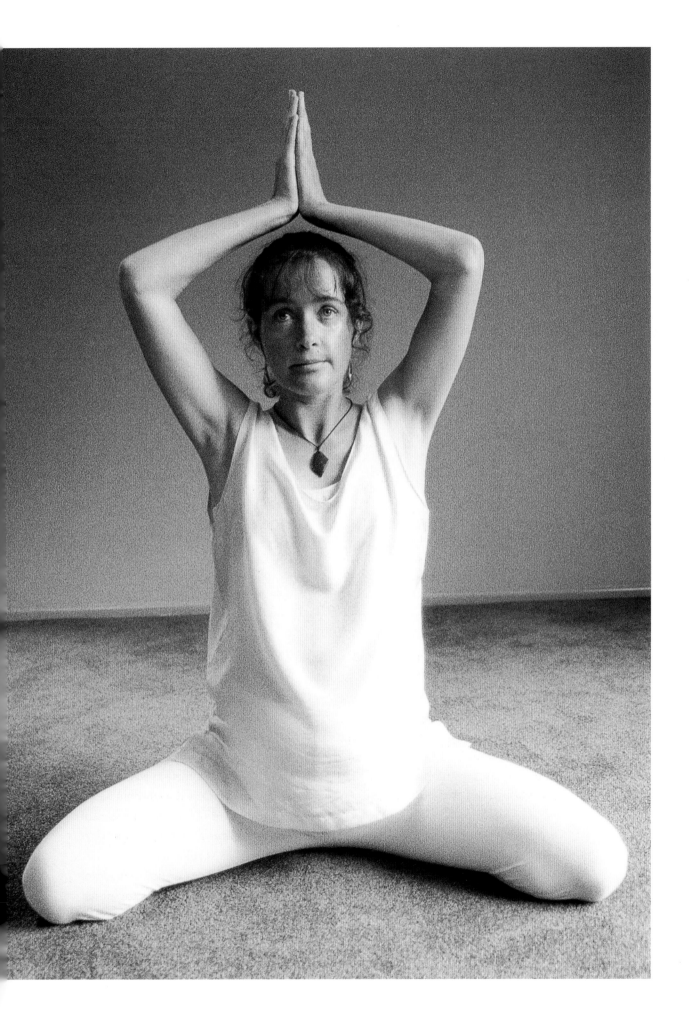

1. From a seated position bend your left arm up behind your back, taking your hand as high up the centre of your back as is comfortable.

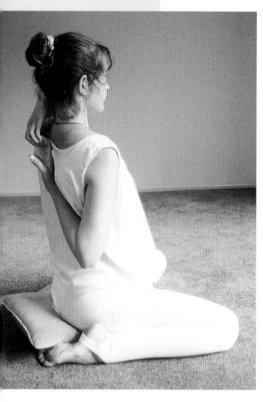

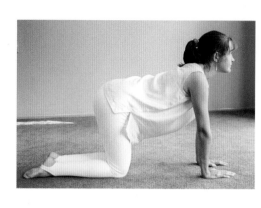

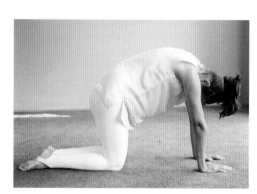

2. Raise your right arm above your head and then take it over your right shoulder towards the fingers of your left hand, joining your fingers if possible. Hold your right arm in an upright position so that your elbow is pointing straight up and your upper arm is beside your ear. If you find that your fingers don't meet, a piece of string or rope can be used to fill the gap until your fingers touch.

3. Once your fingers are together or joined by rope, relax your shoulders and arms and breathe naturally. Remain in this position until you feel an increased warmth in your upper arm.

4. Lower your arms and shake them a little before repeating the exercise with your right arm up the middle of your back.

13. The Cat
(marjariasana)

The Cat is a noteworthy pose to practice throughout pregnancy, with only a slight variation from the traditional posture. The 'all fours' position is particularly comfortable during pregnancy, as the weight is taken away from your pelvic region relieving that heavy feeling often felt during the last trimester. Many women find the hands and knees position is a very comfortable way to be for the contractions, especially in the second stage of labour. If this is the case, it is ideal to relax into the Pose of the Hare when the contraction has finished, to rest and restore energy before the next contraction.

The Cat is especially good for your back, abdomen and pelvis. Stiffness in your back is relieved as the Cat exercises your back from the neck through to your tail bone. Your pelvis is rocked forward and back which will tone the muscles and ligaments of that area and work deeply into your reproductive system. Your whole internal body is toned and your uterine muscles are massaged gently by the alternating movements.

The Cat is well known to relieve general discomfort in your back as well as lower back pain, especially during the last trimester of pregnancy. It is also a useful exercises if you suffer from groin pain in the last weeks before delivery.

38

The complete book of
yoga and meditation
for pregnancy

The 'all fours' position encourages deep breathing which ensures a good oxygen flow to your whole body

.

Caution: Due to the extra weight in your abdominal area during pregnancy, it is important not to curve your back in position 1, as is the case in the traditional pose. During pregnancy, it is necessary to keep your back straight when inhaling so as to lessen any strain on the ligaments of your back. This is in contrast to the traditional position, where your back is deeply curved as your abdomen drops and your back is worked more deeply.

Also, in position 2 where your back is arched upwards, it is not recommended to contract your abdominal area tightly while exhaling. By practising the Cat gently and slowly, your whole spinal column and pelvic area will be massaged, toned and made wonderfully flexible.

1. Come into the 'all fours' position with your knees the same distance apart as your hands and shoulders.

2. Hold your back straight and breathe in, looking straight ahead.

3. Breathe out as you arch your spine so your tail bone is tucked under and your chin comes close into your chest, remembering to keep your arms straight throughout the exercise.

4. Breathe in as you straighten your back. Continue on with these movements up to nine times. When this is completed relax into the Pose of the Hare with your knees wide.

14. The Tiger
(vyaghrasana)

The Tiger is a similar posture to the Cat and it usually follows on from that posture. The benefits are

comparable to the Cat, only in the Tiger you will receive an added stretch in your hip and lower back by extending your leg. This is recommended as an ideal exercise for the relief of sciatica pain which is often a problem during pregnancy. Some people find the Tiger more strenuous than other exercises, so care needs to be taken not to go beyond your own level of fitness. I usually recommend practising between three and five movements on each side, as this will work sufficiently into your hip and your leg.

1. From the 'all fours' position breathe in as you raise your right leg up behind you as high as possible. Lift your head slightly as you look up. Some people like to straighten their leg in this elevated position but your leg can also be slightly bent.

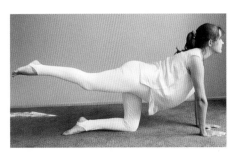

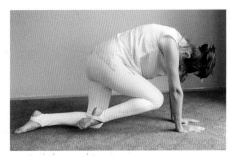

2. Breathe out as you bend your knee, bringing it in towards your face. Your back will be arched as it was for the Cat posture and you will notice a gentle compression in your abdominal area.

3. Breathe in to lift your right leg again and continue on as described, repeating this up to five times with your right leg. Rest if you need to before repeating the Tiger five times with your left leg.

4. When you have completed each side, relax into the Pose of the Hare.

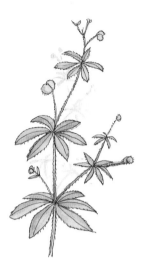

Pelvic Floor Exercises

The importance of the Pelvic Floor exercises during pregnancy and after birth cannot be underestimated. The demands on the muscles and ligaments of the pelvic floor are far greater during pregnancy and childbirth than at any other time in a woman's life but it also needs to be remembered that the pelvic floor plays an equally important role after the birth and that the exercises can restore firmness and strength to the area. In fact, all women of all ages should be aware of supporting the pelvic floor throughout life by practising these simple exercises on a regular basis.

The pelvic floor is a layer of overlapping and interconnecting muscles which extend from your pubic bone at the front to your tail bone at the back and across the seat of your pelvic bone from one side to the other. Within this floor of muscles there are three openings that lead to your pelvic organs; at the front is your urethra which leads to your bladder, your vagina is in the centre leading to your uterus, and your anus is at the back and leads to your rectum and large intestine. These muscles help to support your pelvic organs and your abdominal organs, especially during pregnancy when the weight on these muscles is greatly increased. Also within your pelvic floor muscles are the sphincters, or ring-shaped muscles, of your bladder and your bowel. The purpose of the sphincters is to help control your bowel during bowel movements and the flow of urine when your bladder needs to be emptied. If your pelvic floor muscles are weak, or if these sphincters have lost their elasticity, incontinence can occur.

During the delivery it is important to know how to control these muscles so they can be relaxed and contracted when required. The more relaxed these muscles are, the easier the

40

The complete book of
*yoga and meditation
for pregnancy*

delivery will be and the less chance there is of tearing. The incidence of uterine prolapse is increased when the muscles and the sphincters are lacking tone and firmness. Obviously, the more children a woman has the greater care she will need to take so that the pelvic floor muscles stay firm and elastic throughout her life.

The pelvic floor exercises will help support and tone deeply into your vaginal and cervical areas. They also tighten your anal muscles, which will assist in preventing such problems as constipation and haemorrhoids. They help to prevent the possibility of prolapses occurring either in your anal or uterine areas. The subject of prolapses is not often broached but once they occur they can be very difficult to reverse so it is important to think about prevention early in life and avoid such problems later on.

Unfortunately, in the past it was lack of knowledge and education which contributed to the development of these problems during the child bearing years. There is a natural tendency to bear down during labour and also when emptying your bowels and bladder which over time causes a weakening in this area. Today, the situation is addressed at antenatal classes and there is more open discussion amongst women and between women and their doctors.

Another important topic not discussed enough, is mild incontinence after the birth. This can be extremely distressing and embarrassing. A weakness in your pelvic floor can go unnoticed until you sneeze, cough or even laugh, and is at its worst when you go for a run or do an aerobics class! If you notice yourself already weak in these areas, continued practice will soon rectify the problem.

The pelvic floor exercises are simple enough to do, and can be practised at any time without anyone knowing you are doing them. For example, when you are stopped at a red traffic light or when you are watching a movie you can practise your pelvic floor exercises. If you can make a conscious effort to do them at specific times of the day you will soon enjoy an increased strength, firmness and support.

Some people find it difficult to know when they are actually contracting the pelvic floor muscles and if the lift is enough. To overcome this it is often suggested that you stop the flow of urine mid flow when emptying your bladder. It is your pelvic floor muscles that are being contracted when you do this. By trying this you will know you are using the correct muscles.

1. To practise the pelvic floor exercises sit in a comfortable chair or on the floor with your body relaxed. Gently tighten and hold your whole perineum or pelvic floor. Lift deeply enough to feel this in your bladder without contracting your abdomen. Hold the contraction to the count of five, and then slowly release. This can be repeated as many times as you like or, as a general guideline, practise contracting your muscles nine times, three times a day. This will very quickly tone your pelvic floor.

2. These exercises can also be practised in conjunction with your breathing by contracting your pelvic floor while breathing in then releasing the hold while you breathe out.

Moola bandha

In many ways, the pelvic floor exercises can be loosely compared to the yoga practice of *moola bandha*, which involves lifting, locking and tightening the muscles of your pelvic floor.

Traditionally, *moola bandha* was included in more advanced yoga practices in association with *pranayama* and awareness of the *chakras*.

The word, *moola*, when translated from Sanskrit means root or source. *Bandha* means to lock or tighten a specific part of your body. The nature of the practice is to lift, tighten and hold the muscles of your pelvic floor. When *moola bandha* is practised it is stimulating the base or root *chakra*, known as *mooladhara*, which is said to be located in your perineum. However, to be more accurate, it is the perineum of a man and the cervical area of a woman. I feel when compared to the pelvic floor exercises that the similarities, benefits and applications cannot be overlooked.

In some texts, however, it is *ashwini mudra* which is likened to the Pelvic Floor exercises. I feel that the pelvic floor exercises are, in fact, a combination of *moola bandha* where your cervical area is involved and *ashwini mudra* where your anus is locked. For more details on *ashwini mudra* refer to the chapter, 'Mudras for Pregnancy'.

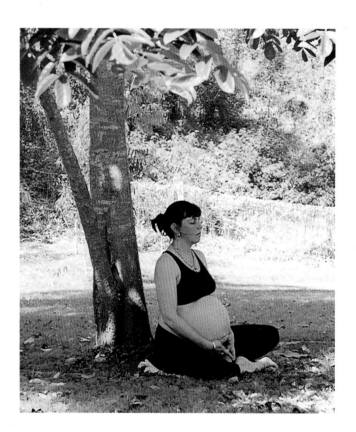

42

The complete book of
yoga and meditation
for pregnancy

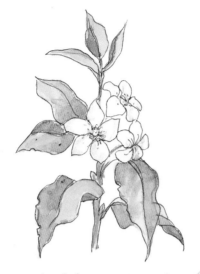

Leg and Abdomen Exercises

Leg & Abdomen

This group of exercises play a significant role in preparing for pregnancy and birth in that they help women to become toned and firm in the legs and abdomen. This helps during pregnancy, delivery and after the birth. They are an essential part of the pregnancy yoga program and can be safely practised throughout the whole pregnancy.

The leg exercises will stretch, tone and greatly strengthen your legs which is very important for increasing stamina and endurance during labour. Many women have commented to me on how strenuous and exhausting labour can be and how important it is to be reasonably fit before that time arrives. Others mention that their legs were sapped of all energy for weeks after the birth, especially if they had a long or particularly arduous labour. Your legs need to be strong if you plan to squat or be in an assisted squatting position during labour. If they are not, they will

feel weak and wobbly and tire quickly.

The leg exercises will also help to relieve backache, mobilise your hips and tone your pelvic area. As your leg muscles are connected to your lower back and pelvic muscles it is important to exercise all these parts of your body. Exercising one area will give strength and tone to the other areas.

The leg exercises can be practised in a continuous flow where one follows the other. Lying on one side of your body you can complete the whole set and then repeating them lying on the other side. By doing this you will not be rolling over from one side to the other after each exercise.

The gentle abdominal exercises will build up and strengthen your abdominal and uterine muscles without causing any strain to your abdominal area. At the same time they will give support and assistance to the muscles of your lower back. Regular practise of the abdominal exercises will keep these muscles in good shape throughout your pregnancy, while your usual firmness and shape will be more easily recovered after the birth.

1. Single Leg Lifts

1. Lie on your right side with your body straight and with your head resting on your right arm or with your arm bent and your head on your hand. Place your left hand on the floor in front of your body to help you remain balanced.

While practising the single leg lifts, keep your knee and foot facing to the front rather than turning your leg to face upwards. You will not lift your leg as high from this position but you will be working your outer thigh muscles and hip, which is the object of this particular exercise. Your inner thigh muscles and your hamstrings will be strongly worked in the following two exercises.

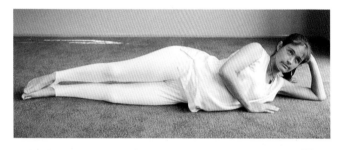

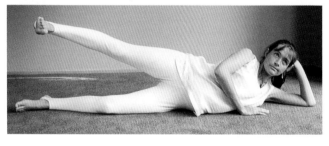

2. Inhale as you slowly lift your left leg.

3. Exhale to lower your leg again.

4. Repeat this movement slowly five or six times. On the last lift, hold your leg in the elevated position, breathing gently, with your awareness on your hip and outer leg. It is

important not to lift your leg more times than you comfortably can, and only hold your leg in the elevated position if you are free of strain or fatigue. Although this is quite a simple posture to do, it is also strenuous and care needs to be taken not to overexert yourself.

5. When you have completed the exercise rest on your back with your knees bent or with your knees tucked into your chest. Be sure you have completely recovered from this exercises before continuing on.

2. The Infinite Pose
(anantasana)

Many yoga postures are named after Hindu gods, or are words of holy reference from ancient Hindu mythology. *Ananta*, when translated, is the name given to Vishnu who was the second deity of the Hindu Trinity. According to legend, he was the preserver of the world. It is also the name given to Vishnu's couch, Sesa, a serpent with a thousand heads which Vishnu rested upon in the primeval ocean. From Vishnu's naval grew a lotus flower from where the first deity of the Hindu trilogy, Brahma – the supreme being and creator of the world, was born. In the southern Indian city of Trivandrum, there is a temple dedicated to Lord Anata Padmanabha and this posture can be seen in that temple. Padma means lotus and nabha means navel.

1. Lie on your right side as for the previous postures. Bend your left leg and hold onto the inside of your left foot with your left hand.

2. Extend your leg fully so that it is straight, stretching deeply into your hamstrings and inner thigh muscles. If you are unable to straighten your leg, hold onto your lower leg or ankle so

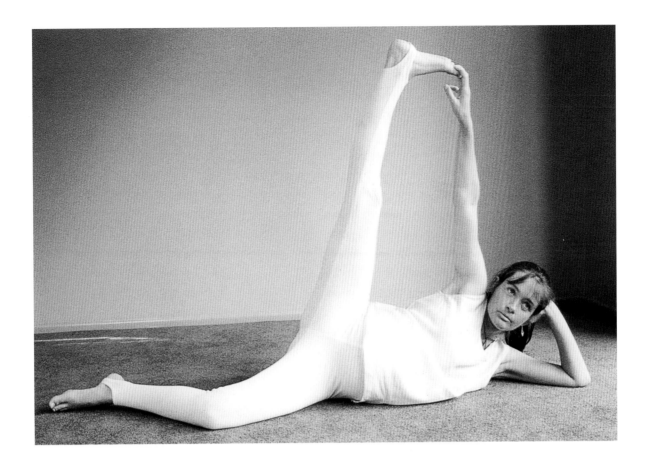

that your leg remains straight. Hold the posture and breath quietly as you relax into the stretch.

Sometimes balancing on the side of your body can be difficult. To overcome this, bend the leg which is on the floor, in this case your right leg, to give you better balance and support.

3. Repeat this posture with your right leg raised.

3. Single Leg Lifts lying on your back

1. Lying on your back with your left leg bent and your right leg straight. The purpose of bending your leg is to prevent any arching or strain to your lower back, and to ensure that your abdominal muscles are doing the work rather than the muscles of your back. Place your hands either under your hips or at shoulder height along the floor with your palms facing down. Some women find it helpful to place a pillow or small cushion under the buttocks for

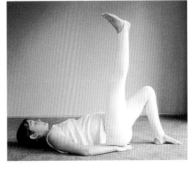

any exercises where they are required to lay on the back.

2. Breathe in as you slowly raise your right leg up as high as possible, keeping your leg straight and your foot relaxed.

3. Breathe out as you lower your leg to the floor.

4. Repeat this five times. Change legs and repeat the exercise five times with your left leg. Keep the middle of

your back flat on the floor. Do not allow an arch or space between your back and the floor. This exercise involves your leg as well as your abdominal muscles so both parts of your body are being exercised and toned.

To work more deeply into your abdominal muscles, only raise your leg half the height of the full extension. Beyond this point it is your thigh and hip muscles which take over. When your hands are placed on your abdomen you can easily feel the muscle groups that are working, especially when your leg is at half height compared to the full extension.

4. Gentle Abdominal exercises lying on your back

Chin to chest exercise

1. Lie on your back with both knees bent and your hands resting on your abdomen.

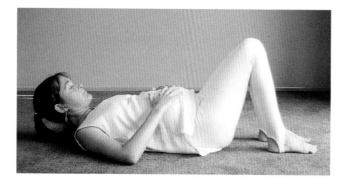

2. As you breathe in, raise your head from the floor, bringing your chin into your chest.

3. Breathe out while lowering your head to the floor. Rest. Repeat this up to nine times without straining the muscles of your neck or your abdomen.

This is a very effective way to tone and strengthen your abdominal muscles and also your neck muscles. It can be safely practised throughout your

pregnancy and quite soon after the birth if the delivery was natural and if your doctor approves.

Single leg bicycles

These exercises can safely be practised during pregnancy to strengthen and tone your abdominal and thigh muscles.

1. Begin by lying on your back with both legs bent and your feet flat on the floor. Your hands are either at shoulder level along the floor, resting on your abdomen or palms down under your buttocks.

2. Make large, slow, circular

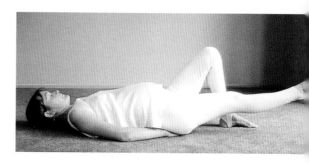

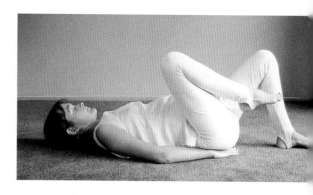

pedaling movements with your right leg, breathing in as your knee is bent and breathing out as your leg is straightened. For the best results bring your knee as close to your abdomen as possible and close to the floor when your leg is straight.

3. Repeat this five times forward and five times backwards.

4. Rest before proceeding with your left leg.

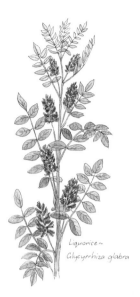

Liquorice~
Glycyrrhiza glabra

Floor Postures and Exercises

Before commencing these exercises it is important to loosen and free your body with a selection of practices from the chapter, 'Warming Up'. If you do this before you begin the floor exercises, you will not be at risk of injury due to cold and tight muscles, and you will receive more benefits from the time you spend doing them.

Always keep in mind that there is no need to compare yourself with others or find fault in your own achievements and remember to relax and enjoy. When yoga is approached in a rigid manner, you are likely to find yourself becoming stiff or sore and your time spent doing yoga could become an ongoing personal battle rather than a pleasure.

Yoga is not a struggle or contest with the self but an opportunity to experience the postures for all their grace at your own pace and within the limits of your ability. When you are practising a posture and are able to

accept your capabilities and limitations exactly for what they are you will also be able to accept that in time your body will gradually unfold to enjoy more flexibility and freedom of movement and therefore you will benefit more from yoga.

1. Closing the Gate
(parighasana)

This is also called the Side Bend on the Knee exercise. Of all the side bending postures, this one will probably give you the most effective extension through the sides of your body. It also deeply stretches the muscles of your inner thigh. As with all yoga postures, it is important to have your whole attention on how you are feeling in the final posture. At no time should you overextend yourself when practising a posture. This is especially important with this exercise due to the extent of the stretch. If you are unable to stretch with your arm lying close to the side of your face, extend your arm upwards instead.

As your body bends to the right, you will notice a strong stretch along the left side of your body, especially in your hip and waist. You will also feel a full extension in your left shoulder and arm, right through to your fingertips. The right side of your body is gently squeezed at the waist, which will work on the organs on that side of your body, such as your liver and the right side of your bowel, gently stimulating and massaging through that area.

Alternatively, when you bend to the left, your pancreas, spleen and the left side of your bowel are benefited. The inner thigh muscles receive a full stretch, the pelvic area is toned and stiffness is removed from your spine and hip. Because of its action on the colon and the liver, this is a very useful posture for the health of your bowel.

Note: Often the tendency is to lean slightly forward with the other shoulder as you bend to the side. The result is that you will extend further but not directly to the side and you will not be in a true side bending posture.

1. From a kneeling position extend your right leg out to the side, making sure that your right foot is in line with your left knee. The right foot is usually placed flat on the floor but, if you prefer, you can have your heel on the floor with your toes turned upwards. Make sure that your right leg is not so far out to the side that your left leg is out of line with that side of your body.

2. Breathe in and raise your arms out to the sides, at shoulder height.

3. Breathe out as you bend your body to the right, resting your right hand on your leg for support. Your right ear, right shoulder and right knee should be in line.

4. Lift your left arm up. If possible, stretch your arm along the side of your face with the palm facing down. Look straight ahead and breathe into the posture for up to nine breaths.

5. Breathe in as you return to the upright position with your arms at shoulder height. Breathe out as you lower your arms.

6. Repeat the exercise to the left.

2. The Crescent Moon
(ardha chandrasana)

When translated, *ardha* means half and *chandra* is moon. *Ardha chandrasana* is a posture resembling a half or a crescent moon. This lovely posture is extremely beneficial for giving tone and strength to your hips, pelvis and upper thigh muscles, while your inner thigh muscles are stretched when your leg is extended back in the full posture (iii).

Caution: The third posture is only suitable for those people who have completed (i) and (ii) easily and with complete comfort.

The full Crescent Moon posture is an intense and dynamic yoga posture and it is important to take care not to overextend yourself. For your added comfort I recommend a small cushion be placed under your knee to help protect your kneecap from strain, especially if you have had a knee injury or if the floor is very hard.

I will detail the Crescent Moon in three stages so that you are able to move gradually from one posture to the next. By evaluating how you feel in posture (i) and (ii) you can consider attempting posture (iii) when you are confident that your body is fully prepared and that you are stretched and toned enough to do so.

48

The complete book of
yoga and meditation
for pregnancy

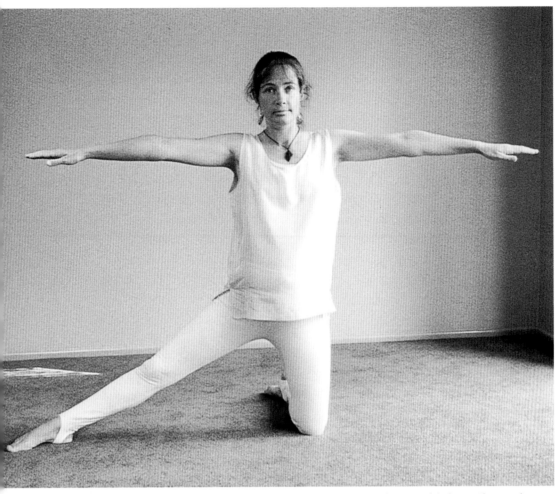

Above and below: Closing the gate

Posture (i)

1. Kneeling on your left knee (with a small cushion under the knee), bend your right knee and place your right foot flat on the floor. Have your right leg far enough forward to feel balanced and steady in this posture.

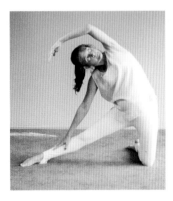

2. The first movement is actually the Equestrian Pose, where your body is stretched forward with your weight over your right thigh and your hands resting on the floor either side of your right foot. As you move forward, have your right knee under your armpit. Your left leg is extended and stretched back. From this posture you will feel a deep expansion throughout your thigh, hip and pelvis.

If your right heel comes away from the floor while lunging forward, your foot needs to be placed further forward before you begin.

3. Relax into the posture and hold it for up to nine breaths or for as long as you are comfortable. When you first practise the Crescent Moon, only hold the final positions for two or three breaths so as to avoid any strain or discomfort.

4. Inhale as you return to the upright position. You may like to relax into the Pose of the Hare before changing sides.

5. Repeat this with the left leg to the front.

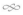

Note: An alternative arm position is to place both hands on the inside of your foot, rather than on either side, especially in the last weeks of your pregnancy when your size might prevent you from placing your hands on either side of your foot.

Posture (ii)

1. From posture (i) straighten your spine so that your arms are resting beside your body. Depending on the length of your arms, you will either find your fingertips reaching the floor, or if not, place

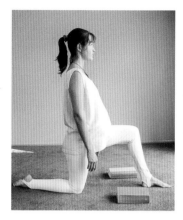

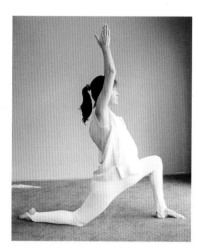

your hands on two stacks of books of equal height, or something else of the correct height so you are able to remain in position without leaning forward. Make sure your back and shoulders are completely relaxed.

2. Breathe quietly while holding this posture, being aware not to experience any strain or difficulty.

3. Inhale as you return to the upright position. Repeat the posture with your left leg to the front.

Posture (iii)

1. Prepare to complete the full Crescent Moon, from posture (ii).

2. When you feel relaxed with the degree you are stretching and can comfortably hold the posture without straining your body, raise both arms above your head with your palms joined, your shoulders relaxed and your elbows straight. In this posture you might imagine you are in a lovely curved arch, like a crescent moon. Stretch from your fingertips, throughout your back, to the toes of your extended foot. Look straight ahead as you breathe naturally and relax deeply into the final posture without strain.

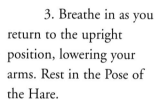

3. Breathe in as you return to the upright position, lowering your arms. Rest in the Pose of the Hare.

4. Repeat the full Crescent Moon posture with your left leg forward.

3. The Seated Triangle
(pavistha konasana)

This is also known as the Wide Leg Stretch and is one of the exercises that can be practised while lying on your back with your legs up against a wall. I mention this now because some women either find it difficult sitting in the wide leg stretch with their back straight or have back and hip problems, which make it unsuitable for them. Also, it is quite common to develop lower back problems or sciatica during the later part of pregnancy in which case I do not recommend this exercise be done from the seated position but rather practise it lying on your back with your legs up a wall. Full details of this procedure are discussed in the chapter 'Squatting'.

50

The complete book of
**yoga and meditation
for pregnancy**

As your pregnancy progresses, you will notice your body becoming looser and more supple. This makes the Wide Leg Stretches easier and more pleasurable to practise due to the extra freedom of movement and flexibility.

It is important to remember not to push yourself into the full posture or to overextend, as it is easy to injure yourself when the posture is not approached in a gentle way. Spend a little extra time, using your breath and your awareness to ease and extend into the posture, staying as relaxed as possible to prevent any tension building up in your body. When your mind and body are free from struggle and there is the least resistance, you are more likely to notice positive results from your yoga.

To relieve strain in your lower back – and for extra support – this posture can be practised resting your lower back up against a wall. Alternatively, place a small cushion under your buttocks to slightly elevate your pelvis and tilt it forward.

With your legs in the wide leg position, the inner thigh muscles receive a deep and full stretch, therefore toning the muscles of your inner thigh and pelvis. The function of the whole pelvic region and the corresponding organs is greatly improved. These exercises have special advantages for pregnant women, even if you only spend time in the upright seated position. When your body is stretched forward between your legs, the whole of your back is stretched, especially across the lower back and hips, and your abdomen and pelvis are gently compressed and massaged.

For those women who are carrying high or who are shorter in the body than others, the forward bending position might become uncomfortable in the last few weeks of pregnancy

because of lack of room. In this case, stretching to the side is the alternative position.

When the stretch is taken over the right and left legs, the major organs of digestion are stimulated and the spinal nerves benefit from a renewed blood flow. Also, as your head is down in the forward bend and side stretches, your mind becomes quiet and calm giving you the opportunity to breathe and relax into the posture.

I feel the most benefits are received from all the forward bending postures when the final position is held for an extended period, allowing the body plenty of time to relax into the stretch. This will give the associated muscles the opportunity to adjust and extend gradually and gently, without resulting in unnecessary strain or tension.

When you first sit in the wide leg stretch, spend some time flexing your feet and pointing your toes to stretch your calf muscles and loosen your ankles.

Stretching forward

1. Sit with your legs as wide apart as possible, your spine straight and your shoulders relaxed. Breathe in and feel as if you are lifting your body upwards from the base of your spine.

2. Breathe out as you bend forward from your waist. Keep your shoulders and arms loose and relaxed and your elbows slightly bent. This will prevent tension being held in your shoulders and upper back. Rest your hands on the floor in front of you and relax your head and neck. While holding this posture, release any tightness in your body and breathe quietly into the stretch. At no time strain or force yourself forward but instead use your breathing and your

Asana
Floor postures and exercises

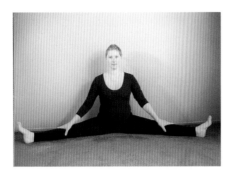

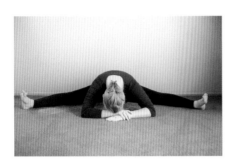

awareness to ease as far into the posture as possible. The more time you spend breathing into the posture and concentrating on releasing tightness and discomfort, the deeper you will go and the more relaxed you are going to feel.

Some women will find they are able to stretch forward easily, resting their elbows and head on the floor. Others will find they can only stretch forward a short way. How far you move forward into the stretch is not relevant to the benefits you will receive from this posture. What is important, is your overall approach when in the posture, how you are feeling in your body, where your thoughts are at the time, and that your awareness is on breathing in a steady and relaxed manner. It is important to realise and accept that we are all built differently. Some women are very supple and have great freedom of movement while others seem tight and less flexible.

Of all the yoga postures recommended, the wide leg stretches reveal more than most about how tight some muscles are and also how uncomfortable a new posture can be. In this exercise we are endeavouring to move the body in ways that are not common to our usual way of being. It is only natural to feel a little awkward to begin with. Try not to be discouraged if you do not make much impression when practising this posture. The

purpose is to stretch and tone your body to your own level of flexibility in a gentle and relaxed way. Wherever you find yourself in the final posture is perfect for you, and from that position you will be receiving all the available benefits. I feel it is important to remember that when you are practising yoga for the first time you are probably using muscles you didn't realise you had and some of them are likely to be tight.

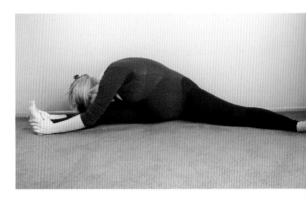

Stretching over each leg

1. From the wide leg position turn your body to the right. Breathe in and stretch your arms above your head, stretching the spinal column.

2. Breathe out and stretch your body out along your right leg. Rest your hands on your leg with your arms slightly bent and bring your head down towards your knee. Take special care that your arms and shoulders are not tense. Only come forward to a position where you can hold the posture in a relaxed manner without bending your knee. Feel the deep stretch throughout your back, in the side of your body and in the hamstrings and thigh muscles. If there is any strain, ease out of the posture slightly. Hold the final posture for nine breaths.

3. Breathe in as you return to the seated position. Repeat the posture, stretching over your left leg.

After spending time relaxing into the forward stretch, you might like to include the following variation. As you

The complete book of
yoga and meditation
for pregnancy

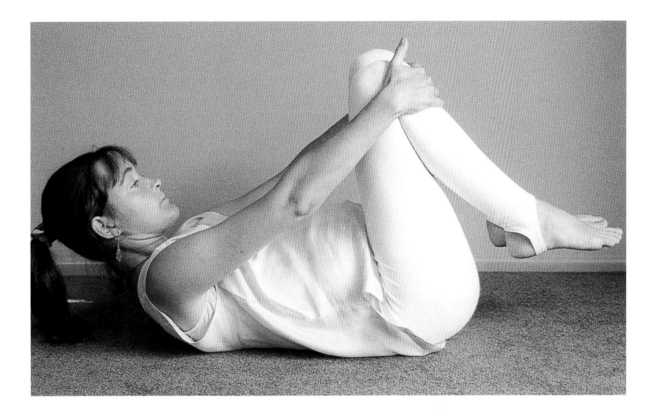

breathe in deeply, lift your body up about half way and then lower yourself back down over your leg as you breathe out. This encourages deeper breathing but also places emphasis on relaxing more fully into the final posture as you breathe out.

Note: When the forward bending postures are completed it is always important to practise a suitable counterpose to relieve your back and to bend your spine the opposite way. You can either lie on your back and bring your knees into your chest, gently rocking your body from side to side, or practise the Pelvis Tilt, the Pose of the Hare or the Cat. Any of these will quickly ease any discomfort in your lower back. A Spinal Twist can also be practised from the wide leg position known as the Dynamic Spinal Twist. Details of this can be found in the chapter 'Spinal Twists'.

4. Churning the Mill
(chakki chalanasana)

This exercise has been modified for pregnancy and is practised from the same wide leg position as the previous posture. It is not a static posture but one where the body is moving from one side to the other so it is a little easier for people to do than the Wide Leg Stretch. Churning the Mill is also included in the 'Postnatal Programs' with a slight variation where the body is taken further back so as to work more deeply into the abdominals. For pregnancy the body is not taken back beyond the upright position.

The same benefits apply for this exercise as for the Wide Leg Stretch but as your body swings freely from the left to the right your waist is also toned. With practise, your hips and spine are loosened and will become more flexible. Tension is relieved in your shoulders and upper back due to the position of your arms.

1. Sit with your back straight and

Practising a counterpose can relieve your back and stretch your spine in the opposite direction

legs as wide apart as possible. For extra comfort place a small cushion under your buttocks or rest with your back against a wall. Lift your arms to the centre front at shoulder height and join your hands together with interlocking fingers.

2. Lean slightly forward and then swing your body out to the right while breathing in.

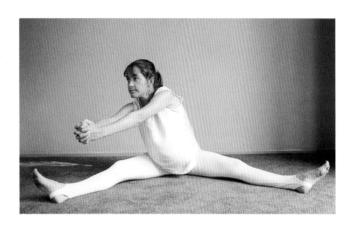

3. Breathe out as you swing your body to the left. The idea is to create a slow, sweeping semicircular movement, moving continuously from the right to the left. Repeat this five times to each side.

4. Bring your legs together when you have completed the posture and shake them lightly.

5. Rowing the Boat
(nauka sanchalanasana)
This is similar to Churning the Mill because it can be modified for pregnancy, yet after the birth it is an excellent posture to practise for its toning effects on the abdominal muscles.

Even in the modified variation, the abdominal muscles are gently toned, which is important for strength and firmness, and the health of the associated organs is also improved. Your hamstring tendons and thigh muscles are stretched as your body is taken

forward and stiffness in your arms and shoulders is relieved.

1. Sit with your legs to the front and your body straight. Join your hands together and lift your arms to shoulder height.

2. Breathe in as you tilt your body back slightly – just beyond the upright position – but without putting any strain on your abdominal muscles. Draw your elbows back and bring your hands into the centre of your chest as if you are rowing a boat.

3. Breathe out as you stretch forward over your legs.

4. Repeat this up to nine times, moving easily and gently forward and back in rhythm with your breathing.

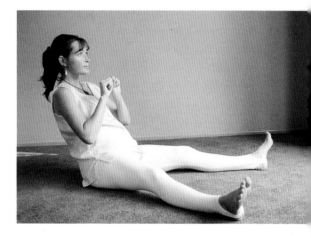

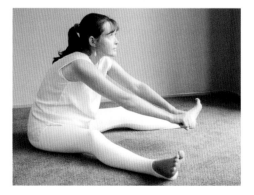

6. Working in pairs from the wide leg position
Working with a partner from the wide leg position often makes this exercise much easier to do and more

The complete book of
yoga and meditation
for pregnancy

enjoyable. It also encourages less resistance and a deeper stretch throughout your inner thighs and back. By working in pairs, there is no need to stretch yourself forward and the result is similar to practising this posture with your legs up against a wall. This method provides an ideal alternative to the Wide Leg Stretch because you are able to relax and ease more gently into the posture. The benefits are similar to practising this posture alone, but there is an added advantage of a deeper stretch throughout the spinal column.

Choose a partner to work with who is about the same height as you and who has similar flexibility. If you find that you are able to spread your legs wider than your partner, ask her to place her feet on the inside of your legs instead of feet to feet. In this way, you will both be able to stretch and extend to your full capacity in complete comfort. Keep in mind that working with a partner for this exercise is meant to make it easier not more difficult, and proper communication is very important. When you communicate with each other you need to build confidence and trust so that both of you know just how far to extend the other. This helps to eliminate any fear of strain or injury.

Bending forward

1. Sit on the floor with your partner and have your legs as wide apart as is comfortable for both of you. Join your feet together and hold hands. It is at this point that any adjustments can be made to your positions.

2. Lean back slightly and gently

ease your partner into the forward bending position. Always communicate with each other so that you are fully aware of how far to move forward into the stretch. When your partner is in the forward stretch make sure she is completely relaxed through her arms and shoulders, that her head is down rather than lifted up, and that she is breathing quietly into the posture. The more emphasis placed on breathing into the stretch, the more beneficial the posture. At no time should either of you overextend yourselves or move beyond a comfortable stretch. The point of this exercise is to have a sense of freedom as you bend forward from your waist.

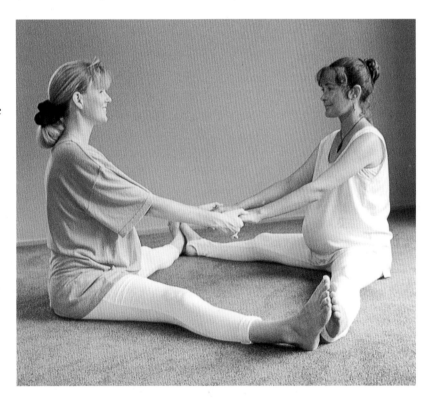

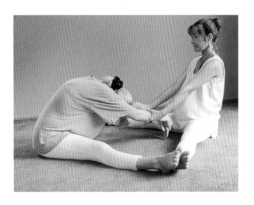

3. Remain in the forward stretch for up to nine breaths before changing roles with your partner. She now stretches you forward.

4. Repeat this exercise three times each side.

Note: If your partner is extremely flexible, hold her by the lower arms or elbows so you don't lean too far back.

Slow circles

This exercise greatly benefits the waist, hips, back, abdominal area and inner thighs. It is very similar to Churning the Mill only with this exercise there is more movement involved as complete circles are made.

1. From the same wide leg position, make slow wide circles with each other, gently leaning back, moving to one side, into the forward stretch

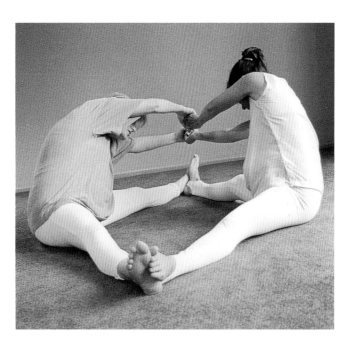

56

The complete book of
yoga and meditation
for pregnancy
∞

posture and then moving to the other side. Make the circles as slow and easy as possible.

2. Continue on in this way – making slow full circles – five times to the right and five times to the left. Try to synchronise the movements with the breathing so that you breathe out as you

move forward and breathe in as you move back.

There seems to be a tendency to speed up when practising these circles, so be conscious of moving slowly. I am sure you will enjoy it much more when it is taken quietly.

7. The Head to the Knee
(janu sirshasana)

When translated from Sanskrit, *janu* means the knee and *sirsha* means the head. The aim of this posture is to bring your head to your knee. This is a graceful yet also challenging posture and there will be some people who find it more difficult to do than others due to the intense stretch in the back and thigh muscles. Rather than forcing your body into the forward bend, it is preferable to be as relaxed as possible and concentrate on gradually easing your body forward without feeling tense or overextending.

When the posture is approached in a relaxed manner and the stretch is within your own level of flexibility, you will find your back muscles, hamstring tendons and thigh muscles lengthening. At no time strain or push yourself beyond comfort, no matter how stiff or flexible you might be.

Wherever you find yourself in the final posture, whether that is stretching easily along the leg or hardly bending forward at all, always be as relaxed as possible and enjoying the posture. More benefits will be achieved by allowing your muscles time to lengthen and gradually ease into the full extension.

Some people are born flexible and can manage many of the yoga positions with effortless ease, whereas others will always find the forward bending postures more difficult to do and quite challenging. However, very often those who find bending forward awkward will discover that the backward bending postures or the spinal twists are more to their liking and easier to so, nature is very kind in this way.

Caution: The forward bending postures have many important benefits to be enjoyed by the majority of women throughout their pregnancies. However, if you are not comfortable it is better to discontinue these exercises in the last few weeks of the pregnancy. Also, if you develop lower back problems during your pregnancy or have other spinal difficulties, proceed very gently or find an experienced teacher who can advise you correctly. If the pain persists, discontinue the practice.

1. Sit on the floor with your legs straight in front of you and your back straight.

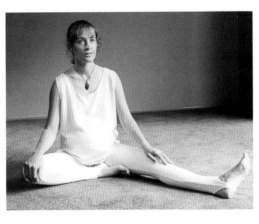

2. Bend your left knee and place the sole of your left foot on the inside of your right thigh.

3. Breathe in and stretch tall throughout your back, lifting from the base of your spine.

4. Breathe out as you bend your body forward, bringing your head as close to your knee as possible. Rest your hands on your foot or on your leg, and bend your arms slightly to prevent any tension forming in your upper back or shoulders. It is better to bend your left arm slightly and rest your hand on your

right leg or knee than to reach for your foot. This will help maintain relaxation in your whole body. When the final posture is held in a relaxed manner, you will feel yourself easing further into it and the muscles of your neck, back and leg gradually being lengthened and freed of tightness. The longer you spend in the posture, the closer you will gradually come to your knee.

5. Hold the posture as you breathe quietly for up to nine breaths. If you have a tendency to bend your knee, lift up a little so that your leg remains straight.

6. Breathe in as you return to the seated position, shaking your legs lightly.

7. Repeat this with your left leg extended to the front.

I have found that the longer you

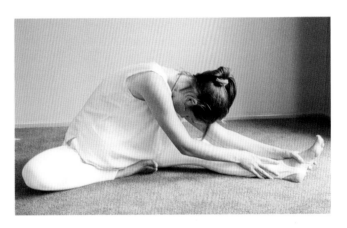

spend in the final posture the more fully your body eases into the stretch. If you are inclined to increase the length of time you spend in this posture, remember to hold the posture for the same number of breaths on both sides.

8. The Pelvic Tilt

The Pelvic Tilt is a modified version of the Shoulder Pose, which is detailed in the section, 'Postnatal Programs'. The only difference between the two postures is that the hips are not lifted as high in the Pelvic Tilt as for the

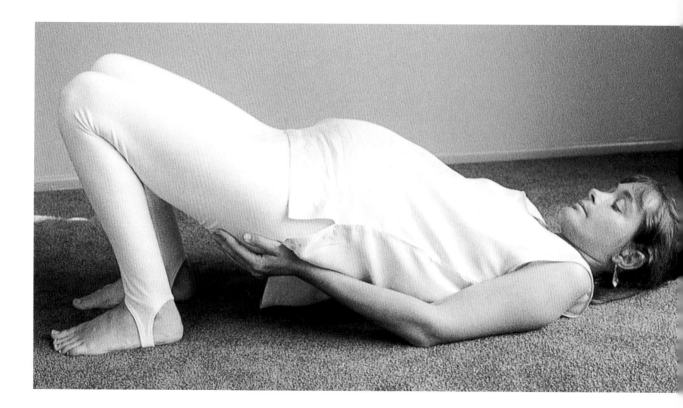

Shoulder Pose making it more suitable for pregnancy.

The Pelvic Tilt has many benefits for pregnant women and has been recommended by well-informed authorities on pregnancy and childbirth. In my experience, there has been no apparent discomfort or contraindications from the Pelvic Tilt and most women seem to enjoy the weight being eased from their lower body. However, if you feel any discomfort or fullness in the face, I recommend you discontinue the exercise.

The Pelvic Tilt is sometimes recommended in cases where the baby is lying transverse or in some situations where the baby is breech. However, the concern in both these situations is that the baby is in those positions for an internal reason and may not be able to come easily into the head down position. I am fully aware this is not always the case and that this is not a medical book, however, I feel it is important to consider why a baby is in

the breech position, before presuming the Pelvic Tilt will rectify the problem. If you know your baby is in either of these positions, always seek professional advice before trying to turn your baby around. It is worth noting that most doctors do not like attempting to turn a breech baby due to the risks involved.

This valuable posture is particularly useful for relieving lower back pain. Pressure in the lower pelvic area and groin is alleviated especially in the last weeks of pregnancy, as the Pelvic Tilt moves the baby higher into the body away from the pelvis.

It has also been recommended as a precautionary exercise against the possibility of hernias due to the fact that your weight is more evenly distributed to the middle of your body. The reproductive area is toned and digestion is improved as pressure on your bowel and the organs of your digestive system is relieved when gravity is reversed.

This is an ideal posture to practise regularly if you have pockets in your large intestine (diverticulitis), haemorrhoids, or a problem with gas. In the final posture your chin is held close to your chest, which has a normalising effect on the thyroid and parathyroid glands in your throat.

1. Lie on your back with your knees bent and your feet a little apart and flat on the floor. Place your feet as close to your buttocks as possible.

2. Breathe in and lift your hips as high as possible, keeping your head on the floor and your chin locked into the chest. Your hands can remain, palms down, on the floor or be placed under your hips for extra lift and support. Your feet can be flat on the floor but if you want more lift in the pelvis rise up onto your toes.

3. Breathe out and lower your hips to the floor.

4. This can be repeated up to five times. As an alternative, you can hold the final posture for longer, while breathing and relaxing.

Note: If the Pelvic Tilt is not a comfortable position for you, a suitable alternative is to lie with the legs up the wall, the knees slightly bent and the feet flat on the wall. Have the buttocks as close to the wall as possible and lift the hips slightly to the desired height. You can also place two or three cushions under your buttocks to give you the same lift and tilt in the pelvis, without the effort of holding your body up yourself. Remain in this position, relaxing into the body with your awareness on the breath. If you are carrying a lot of extra weight and there is a feeling of fullness in the face, I don't recommend this posture be practised in the last month of pregnancy.

9. The Monkey Chief
(hanumanasana)

The Ramayana is an epic tale from ancient India and in it the story of Hanuman, the powerful Monkey chief,

can be found. Hanuman was the son of Anjana and Vayu the god of the winds, and this story reveals how he saved the life of his ailing friend by leaping – in one bound – from Sri Lanka to the Himalayas where he gathered a precious life saving herb. This posture, also known as the Leg Splits, is dedicated to him and that enormous leap.

Certainly, this posture will not interest everyone due to the radical stretch it involves, however, even in a modified form it has many benefits for pregnancy. I will detail it in a much modified form where the body is fully supported but where the benefits will still be apparent to the inner thigh and groin muscles. In this form, *hanumanasana* is suitable for those who wish to include it in their yoga program during pregnancy. It is definitely the most extreme posture I will recommend and, with that thought in mind, it is not suitable for those who are new to yoga or who are tight in their inner thigh muscles.

When *hanumanasana* is practised in its complete form it is a very beautiful, balanced and graceful posture. In this form or to a lesser degree in the modified variation, it will work into the muscles of the legs, the lower back, the pelvis and hips. Circulation is greatly improved to these areas and it is useful in assisting women with sciatic problems. The stretch felt in your legs is quite obvious in both the full stretch and the modified form. The pelvis and hips are also toned and balanced.

Caution: When you are in the modified posture, do not take your hands from the floor but use them as supports while the posture is held. In time, your level of flexibility will increase. Remember that the benefits are there for you no matter how far you extend into the stretch.

1. From a kneeling position extend your right leg out to the front and place both hands on the floor, either side of your left knee.

2. Straighten your knee and very gently and gradually ease your right leg forward, keeping your hands on the floor, until you are satisfied you have stretched to your own level of flexibility. Be careful that you are definitely not straining and most importantly that there is no pain. Come to a position that is suitable for you, where you are obviously aware of stretching but without any discomfort.

3. Hold the final position while you relax and breathe into the posture. If you are in the full split, join the palms of your hands in the centre of your chest.

4. Return to position 1 and repeat the procedure with your left leg forward. Rest and relax after the posture is completed.

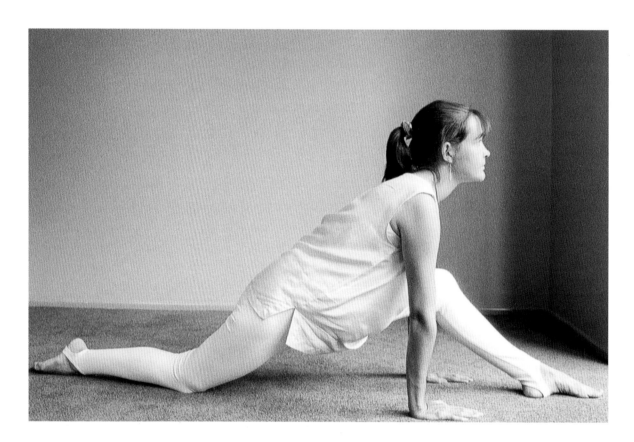

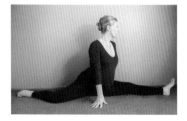

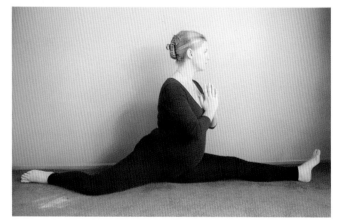

The complete book of
**yoga and meditation
for pregnancy**
∞

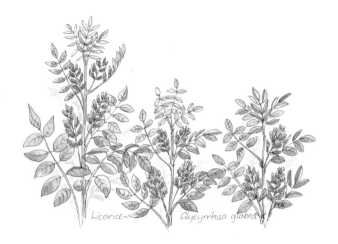

Licorice ~ Glycyrrhiza glabra

Squatting

From Victorian times, women in western countries have been required to deliver from a lying down position. It was considered unnatural and immodest to deliver in any other way, even though this position completely defies gravity and makes a woman's task more difficult. Women today are more fortunate as our comfort and needs are considered very important and there is a greater understanding of the whole birthing process.

Since ancient times squatting has been used for childbirth. Today, in eastern cultures and some Third World countries, the squatting position is still used by many women for birthing. Often the women of these countries give birth from the full squatting posture and apparently with less difficulty than we do in the West. Their deliveries are generally shorter and need less intervention. I am not suggesting that if you squat for delivery it will automatically guarantee your labour will be the easiest but there are many advantages to squatting during delivery.

In New Active Birth, Janet Balaskas (page 14) gave the following important reasons why squatting is recommended – for both mother and baby – during pregnancy and labour.

Squatting is closest to nature's laws and is known as the physiological position. A position is physiologically effective:
- *when there is no compression on the vena cava and the aorta*
- *when the pelvis becomes fully mobilised*
- *Supported squatting seems to be especially efficient at the end of the second stage when the baby is being born.*

The squatting position produces:
- *maximum pressure inside the pelvis*
- *minimum muscular effort*
- *optimal relaxation of the perineum*
- *optimal fetal oxygenation*
- *a perfect angle of descent in relation to gravity*

(Balaskas 1989)

Squatting can also be used as a general sitting position for both working and resting. Small children squat while playing and it is a natural and obviously comfortable position for them to be in. It is not uncommon to see people of all ages in many eastern countries relaxing in a squatting position while sipping tea and sharing conversation with friends. There seems to be no sign of discomfort as people can be seen squatting for hours while in their homes preparing meals, in their shops or working in the fields.

Benefits
- Your uterine and pelvic floor muscles are toned and strengthened.
- The muscles of your thighs, knees, calves and ankles are exercised and your feet are massaged in all the squatting postures. Circulation is greatly improved to your lower limbs and to your pelvic area. Stiffness is removed from your legs and hips.
- Your hips become more flexible and your lower back muscles are toned and stretched. This is particularly important during pregnancy because your lower back often develops a 'sway', causing some women to experience severe pain in that area. The squatting position reduces the curve in your back and relieves pressure on the discs of your spine as your pelvis is tilted upwards. This means that the vertebrae of your lower spine are rounded and flexed, resulting in less strain. Women who are suffering from considerable lower back pain and especially sciatica in the last trimester, gain excellent relief from either the full squatting postures or the modified forms.
- When a woman is in labour in either the squat or a modified squatting posture, her pelvis is closer to being

vertical and the child descending in the birth canal can be delivered more easily. Contractions are often less intense when a woman is in a squatting posture.
- The incidence of uterine prolapse is lessened with regular squatting practise because the pelvic floor and inner thigh muscles are toned and strengthened. These muscles assist in supporting your uterus, bladder and other pelvic organs.
- It is recommended for people who are prone to constipation and haemorrhoids, to practise squatting as regularly as possible. Both of these problems are quite common during pregnancy.
- All the squatting and seated postures help to hold your spinal column straight so that your internal organs are neither cramped or congested. This is important to remember as more efficient circulation is supplied to your abdominal organs.
- Squatting is very beneficial during the second stage of labour as the diameter of your pelvis increases up to 2 cm.

By practising the squatting postures with your partner and birth assistants during pregnancy you will be more familiar with the variations that can be managed comfortably during labour. The more practise you do the easier it will be to sustain these positions in labour. During labour, a squatting-type posture can be arranged where you are fully supported on both sides by people present at the birth.

Although squatting is not always easy to begin with, perseverance and practice are well worth the effort and initial discomfort. For some people it can be quite challenging and often extremely difficult to learn squatting as an adult, but it needs to be remembered

The complete book of
yoga and meditation
for pregnancy

that squatting is a natural and 'possible' position for almost everybody.

Note: Before you begin the squatting exercises, practise the hip rotations and even the Butterfly to loosen your hips in preparation for squatting.

For people who have varicose veins, the moving squat or postures where your body is not stationary will prevent any discomfort from reduced circulation. This also applies to women who have a cervical stitch.

As with all exercises, there are always those who will find the squats to be just not suitable. If you have a serious back injury or problems with your knees you may be better to try a modified form of the full squat.

1. Full squatting and the Moving squat

Full squatting is practised with your feet flat on the floor, your knees wide and your spine straight. If this is too difficult for you when you first attempt squatting, there are a number of alternatives that are quite acceptable.

For example, you can squat with your back leaning against a wall, on your toes rather than with your feet flat on the floor, sitting on a low stool, on a step or on a stack of large books.

The moving squat is where you transfer your weight from one foot to the other in a rocking movement from side to side. This helps your legs to become accustomed to squatting and is recommended if you are unable to stay in the static posture for the reasons mentioned earlier, or if you become too uncomfortable.

1. Stand with your feet about the width of your shoulders apart. Bend your knees and come into a full squatting posture. Keep your arms relaxed and rest your hands comfortably

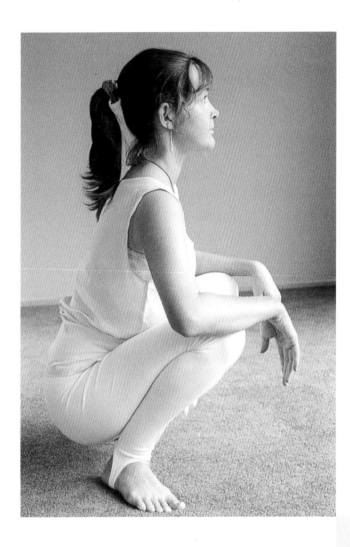

on your knees. Have your knees wide apart and lean your body slightly forward.

2. Remain in the static posture or place your hands on the floor between your feet and move from one foot to the other in a rocking motion. This rocking movement will relieve stiffness and loosen your hips, knees and ankles. The movement will also help you to relax into the posture more easily even if you are familiar with squatting and find it quite comfortable.

3. Relax into the full squatting posture and remember to breathe naturally. When you have held the squat for the desired time, return to a standing position or place your hands behind your back and lower your buttocks to the floor, stretching your legs out in front of you.

4. From either the standing or sitting position, rotate your ankles slowly in both directions and shake your legs lightly.

2. Stretching and Squatting

This posture will give your hips, knees and ankles greater flexibility and is an ideal exercise to do before the other squatting postures. Your legs are alternatively stretched, as one leg is extended to the side while the other is bent. You will observe a deep stretch in your inner thigh area.

1. Begin in the squatting posture either with your feet flat on the floor or on your toes.

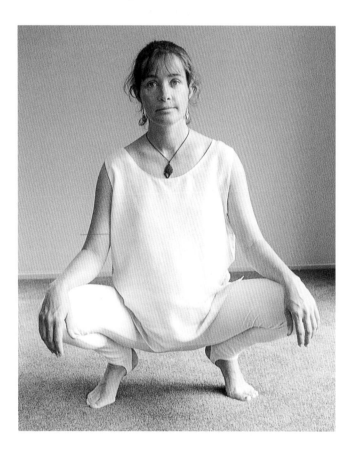

64

The complete book of
yoga and meditation
for pregnancy

2. Place your hands on the floor between your feet. Extend your right leg to the side, keeping your right heel on the floor and your leg straight. Most of your weight will be on your left foot.

3. From this position, place your right foot flat on the floor and transfer your weight from left to right. Extend your left leg to the side. To begin with, you might need to bring your foot in slightly before you move from one foot to the other.

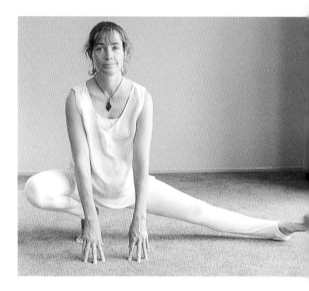

4. When you have the idea of moving freely from one foot to the other, repeat this up to five times each side. Do this slowly, spending some time with your leg to the side so you are able to feel the benefits of the stretch in your inner thigh and the flexion of the hip and knee in your other leg. This is an excellent way to loosen and free your hips in preparation for the other squatting postures.

3. The Salute Squat
(namaskarasana)

For women who enjoy squatting, this lovely posture will supply all the benefits that squatting provides, while at the same time helping to breathe deeply and expand into your groin and pelvic floor.

Although the Salute is traditionally practised with feet flat on the floor, it can also be done on your toes or on a low stool for easier balance and comfort.

1. Begin the Salute from the Full Squat posture. Stretch your arms out

between your legs. Join the palms of your hands together and lower your head down between your shoulders. Be aware that your neck and shoulders are relaxed. The outer part of your upper

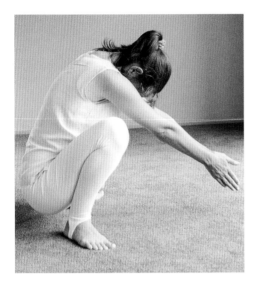

arms and shoulders will be resting on the inside of your knees.

2. Breathe in as your hands are brought, palms together, to the centre of your chest into a prayer position. This movement will cause your elbows to gently push your knees a little wider,

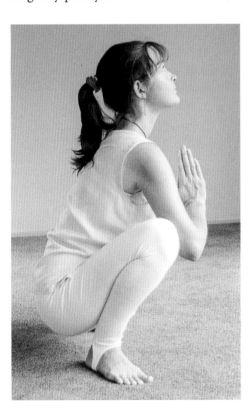

opening up your pelvic area and inner thighs. Straighten your back and look upwards. In this position, you will feel a deep stretch and full expansion in your hips and inner thighs. Deeper breathing becomes possible as your back is straightened and your chest is opened.

3. Breathe out as you extend your arms forward between your knees, lowering your head down between your shoulders.

4. Continue on with both movements of this posture, inhaling as you gently open your knees wider with your elbows and exhaling as your head is lowered.

5. Repeat this up to nine times and then rest in a sitting position with your legs stretched in front of you. Slowly rotate your ankles and shake your legs to relieve any discomfort you might be feeling.

4. Gas Relieving Posture
(vayu nishkasana)

This posture has a very beneficial effect on your whole digestive system and is useful for removing gas and discomfort from your abdominal area. It is recommended as a relief from constipation and haemorrhoids and is an excellent tonic to the nerves of your legs, arms and shoulders. With regular practice this posture will keep your body flexible and loose while also supplying all the other benefits of squatting.

This posture is commenced from a full squat posture, either with your feet flat on the floor or from your toes.

1. From the full squat posture, place your hands on your lower legs or hold onto your big toe with your thumb and first finger.

2. Breathe in as you rise into a bent-over, standing position with your legs straight, holding onto your toes. If

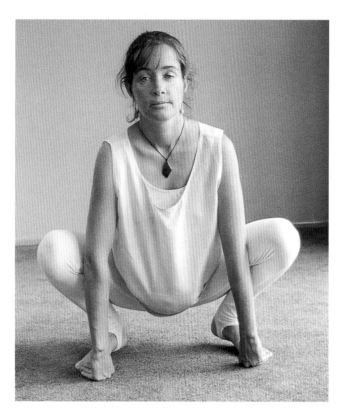

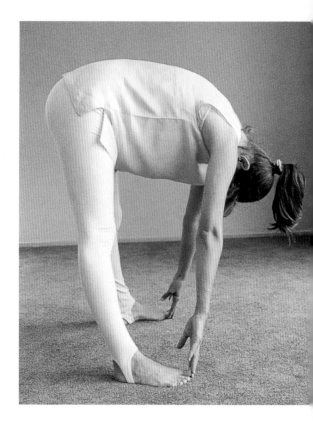

you are unable to reach your toes, hold onto your ankles or lower legs instead.

3. Breathe out as you bring your head in towards your legs, stretching your hamstrings.

4. Breathe in and look up.

5. Breathe out as you come back into the squat posture. The four movements of the squatting and standing exercise need to be coordinated with two full breaths.

6. The movement can be repeated up to nine times. When you have completed the exercise, rest your legs as detailed for the other squatting postures.

5. The Deep Standing Squat
(utthanasana)

Utthanasana is a very important and powerful yoga posture. It strengthens your thighs, buttocks, and, more importantly, the muscles of your lower back. It is quite deceiving because it does not look as strenuous as it really is, and care needs to be taken not to

hold the final posture for longer than is realistic for your level of strength and physical endurance. If you find this especially strenuous, it is better to repeat the exercise more often and remain in the deep squat for a shorter time, until your strength improves. If you begin to feel weak and fatigued while holding the posture, or if your breathing rate increases, come out of the posture immediately and rest until your breathing has returned to normal.

Although this is a strong posture, you will become aware that when it is practised regularly, vigour and tone will be improved throughout your whole body. It is an excellent posture to practise during pregnancy as it helps create the stamina, strength and willpower needed for labour. It is one of the foremost postures to consider if you have a weak lower back.

1. Stand with your feet turned out, about a metre apart. Hold your spine straight and let your arms hang relaxed from your shoulders.

66

The complete book of
yoga and meditation
for pregnancy

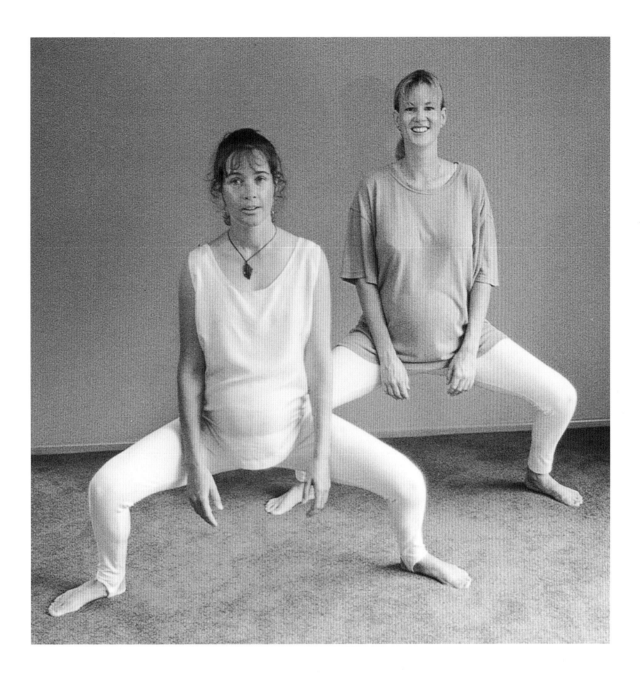

2. Breathe in to prepare and as you breathe out bend your knees and lower yourself into a deep standing squat. Your knees and thighs are open wide so you will experience a deep inner thigh stretch. Lower yourself as deeply into the squat as you are comfortable with and hold that posture. Keep your breathing natural and relaxed. Relax your upper body and hold your back straight. It seems easier to hold the posture when the muscles of your buttocks and pelvic floor are tightened and your pelvis is tilted forward.

3. Breathe in and return to the standing position. Rest and relax before repeating the posture. Each time you repeat the squat, try to move more deeply into it without forcing yourself into a position of discomfort or strain. When you have completed the posture move your feet closer together and shake your legs lightly. If you are quite strong and find this exercise easy, it can be held for longer as long as your breathing is even and relaxed. If you hold this posture for too long you will experience fatigue and weakness.

6. The Deep Standing Squat with a Spinal Twist

This exercise is very relaxing for the back and is particularly good for relieving tightness and stiffness from your spine.

1. From the deep standing squat posture extend your arms out to the sides.

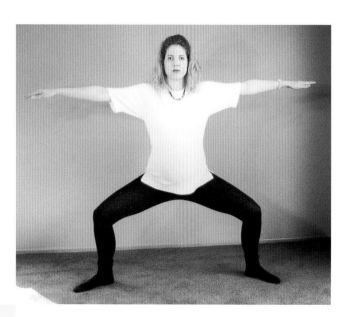

2. Turn your body as far to the right as you can and wrap your arms around your body while looking over your right shoulder.

3. Repeat this movement on the opposite side by swinging to the left in a smooth flowing movement. Repeat up to five times in each direction.

4. When you have completed the exercise return to the centre, lower your arms and come out of the squatting posture. When your body moves from right to left you are no longer in a static squatting posture, which makes it easier to do and to hold for longer.

7. Crow Walking

When I practise this exercise I feel more like a member of the monkey family than a crow, as monkeys and apes take leisurely walks around the forest floor in this manner. The word

'leisurely' is quite important here because this is how I would like you to feel when moving around in the Crow Walk, rather than feeling awkward and uncomfortable which is often the case.

This has not been the most popular of exercises to teach and there are definitely those of you who will object to it quite strongly when it is first

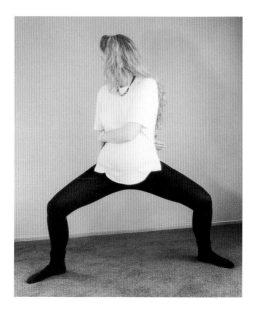

practised. However, I hope that with knowledge of its many benefits you will be encouraged enough to keep practising. I have noticed that pregnant women seem to enjoy this exercises far more than other people and are also more likely to persevere with it.

Crow Walking is an ideal alternative if the static squatting postures are not suitable for you. It has all the benefits of the squatting postures and it is an especially good exercise for overcoming constipation and improving circulation to your feet, legs and pelvic area. Approach this exercise with joy and ease and it will become as pleasurable to do as the other postures. You will notice it is easier to do when you have become more accustomed to the other squatting exercises.

1. Crow Walking is really a continuous walking squat or waddle,

68

The complete book of
yoga and meditation
for pregnancy

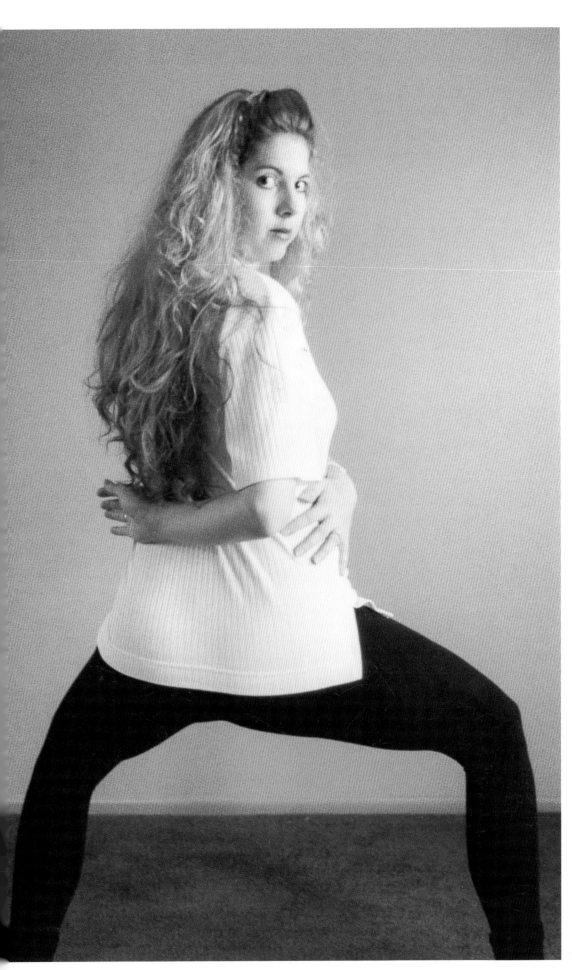

*The Deep
Standing
Squat with a
Spinal Twist*

69

moving slowly forward on your toes, one leg after the other. Start off going only a short distance until you become used to the exercise and then gradually extend the distance over time. When you have walked your desired distance, rest in a sitting position and shake your legs lightly.

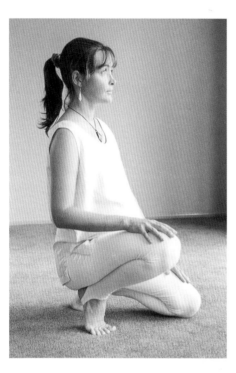

8. Wall Stretches

These are alternative ways to practise the Full Squat, the Butterfly and the wide leg stretches. They are especially good for women who are not comfortable in the seated positions. They are recommended if you have a lower back problem or if the problem is aggravated after practising the individual postures.

Even if you are flexible and enjoy the seated positions, you will feel a much deeper stretch when these three exercises are practised lying on the floor. This is because pressure is taken off your back when you are lying down and gravity is working with you to assist the movement. Lying down will also prevent you from pushing your body

too far into the postures because the weight of your legs and gravity will be assisting you to 'open' more fully.

From the lying position the inner thigh stretch and the depth of tone experienced throughout the pelvic areas is actually more than from the seated position. I have found most pregnant women really enjoy this way of practising and for some it becomes the preferred way of doing them during pregnancy and after the birth.

The wall exercises provide an acceptable way to modify the yoga postures to suit the needs of the individual, without becoming too far removed from the original postures. As with all yoga practices, they are always practiced with full breath and body awareness.

Note: Some women are not comfortable lying on their backs in the last weeks of pregnancy and if this is the case discontinue the exercise immediately.

The easiest way to prepare for the wall stretches is to sit with your left hip against the wall and then lay down on your back as you swing your body around and lift your legs up the wall. Sometimes resting your head on a pillow helps to overcome nausea and discomfort.

The Squat

Lie on your back with your body straight, your buttocks as close to the

The complete book of
yoga and meditation
for pregnancy

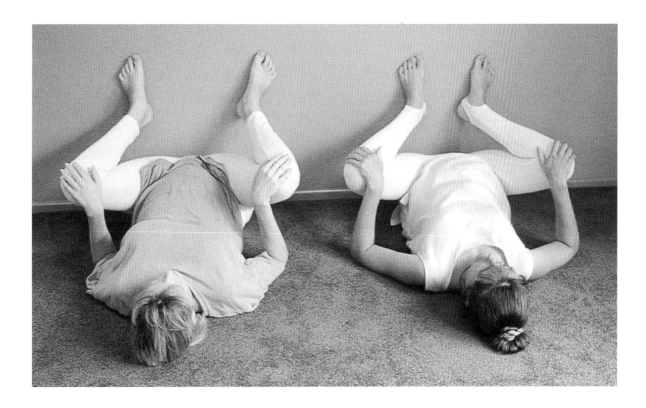

wall as possible and your legs straight up the wall. Separate your feet slightly as you would if you were squatting on your feet and bend your knees so that your feet move close to your buttocks, keeping your heels on the wall.

Rest your hands on your knees and gently open your knees wider, in this way opening up throughout your inner thigh and your pelvic region. Do not force your legs into an uncomfortable position. Remain in this posture while breathing naturally.

The Butterfly

From the same lying down position, bring the soles of your feet together with your knees open wide and your hands resting on your knees. As you breathe out, gently ease your knees open towards the wall, relaxing deeply into the position with each breath. Rest from time to time and try to 'breathe' into the stretch as you imagine your outgoing breath opening your pelvis and inner thighs.

The weight of your legs will assist with opening throughout your pelvic area and all the muscles in this part of your body will be toned and stretched.

The Wide Leg Stretch

Prepare for the Wide Leg Stretch as you have for the Squat and the Butterfly. When you are ready, open your legs as wide as possible, keeping

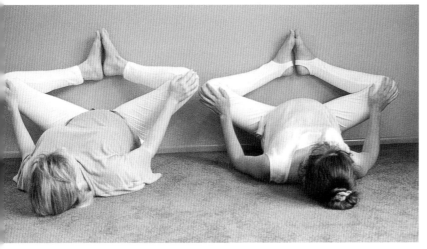

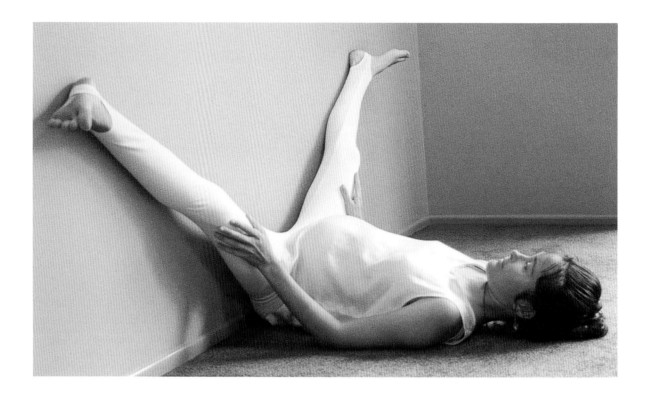

your legs straight and feeling the weight of your legs stretching your inner thighs.

Relax and breathe steadily, holding the posture for as long as you are comfortable. Use your outgoing breath to ease into the position. For

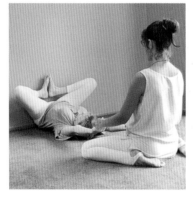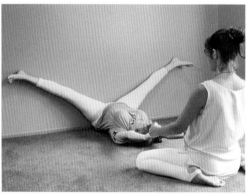

those women who find it a bit squashy bending forward in the last weeks of pregnancy, the wall stretch is an ideal alternative.

Remember also that lying with your legs straight up the wall gives great relief for tired and aching feet and fluid retention in your ankles or feet.

Working in pairs

From any of these positions you can work with a partner for a wonderfully deep stretch throughout your back and spinal column.

Extend your arms along the floor behind your head. Your partner, kneeling behind you, very gently pulls on your arms so as to stretch the whole of your back. It is very important to communicate with your partner at all times, indicating just how far you would like to stretch. At no time should you feel any discomfort, tension or strain in any part of your body.

The aim of this exercise is to be as comfortable as possible while still feeling all the benefits of the posture and the deep stretch through your back. This is a very effective way of stretching and relieving tightness in your upper and middle back.

72

The complete book of
yoga and meditation
for pregnancy

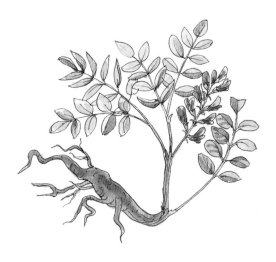

Balancing

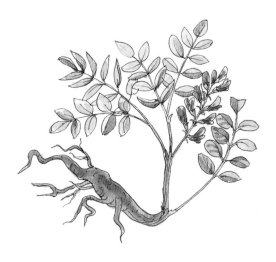

The balancing postures are a very important part of any yoga program. Generally, they are not strenuous or demanding on the body, making them ideal for pregnancy and especially for someone who is a beginner to yoga. I recommend that you include at least one balancing posture in your yoga program, after first warming your body with some gentle stretches.

During pregnancy your whole shape, size and weight are continually changing so it is important to be aware of your posture and carriage. Maintaining correct posture plays an important role in the prevention of backache, especially during the later months. If you look in a mirror side-on, you will notice if you are standing correctly or if you are developing a sway. The more regularly the balancing postures are practised the better your posture will be and the more poise and grace you will maintain.

As your balancing ability improves so will your general concentration and alertness, enabling you to remain focused without your mind wandering. This enhanced alertness and concentration supports a sense of inner calmness. Nervous tension is removed and a feeling of stillness and quietness is experienced. If you were to practise all the balancing postures together, where one posture follows on from another, you would notice all your energies being drawn into a central point of awareness that is steady and focused. This is the same as the feeling experienced during meditation. From this point of view these postures resemble a meditation in movement.

The most difficult aspect of these postures is the ability to stand on one leg with full breath and body awareness, without losing your balance. Any difficulty you might be experiencing can be overcome if you gaze at a stationary object. This will help steady your concentration and prevent you from losing your balance. It is interesting to note that when people forgo their point of focus and start thinking of other things, they often lose their balance. I suggest you also count your breaths as this is an effective way of keeping your mind focused and it helps you to hold the posture for the same length of time on both sides.

Keep the supporting foot and leg relaxed to alleviate any tension and rigidity in your stance. You will also find balancing on one leg easier if your toes are spread evenly across the floor. Gripping the floor with your toes causes tension in the muscles of your feet and results in less contact with the floor.

Some people find it helpful to stand either facing a wall or with their back a few centimetres away from a wall, depending on the posture. This will provide support if you do lose your balance, and can remove the fear of falling. However, within a short space of time you will become steady and be able to stand, unaided, for as long as desired.

1. The Tree
(vriksasana)

The Tree is a classic balancing posture, one that is very simple to do yet full of grace and merit. Physically, your supporting leg becomes stronger, your hip and thigh become more flexible and your knee is 'opened' out to the side.

This posture was practised by the yogis of India thousands of years ago. They were known to stand in this position for many days, deep in

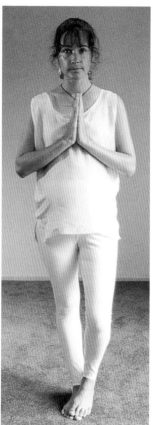

meditation. If you were to visit the holy city of Varanasi, on the sacred Ganges river, you might see this very thing happening today.

1. Begin by standing with your feet a little apart and your body relaxed.

2. Choose a stationary object at eye level to focus on. When you are ready, rest your right foot on top of your left foot. You may wish to remain in this position until you gain confidence and your balance improves before lifting your leg to the traditional

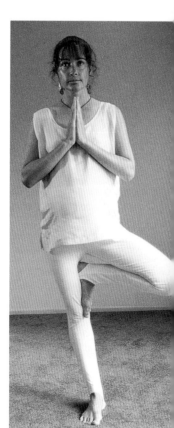

position. The most relevant point of this exercise is to balance on one leg, not where your elevated leg is positioned.

3. Place your right foot high on the inside of your left thigh. Alternatively, if your ankle is supple enough you can place your foot in front of your thigh, in a Half Lotus position. In either of these positions, your knee is taken out to the side, which encourages your hip

to open. You will feel a deep stretch throughout your inner thigh and pelvic area.

4. Join your hands together at the centre of your chest in the prayer position. Keep your shoulders relaxed. Hold the final position for nine breaths. With practice, the Tree can be held for as long as desired.

5. Lower your foot to the floor and lightly shake your legs and feet.

6. Repeat the posture standing on your right leg, remembering always to hold the posture for the same amount of time on both sides.

The Dynamic Tree

The Tree can also be practised with your arms raised above your head.

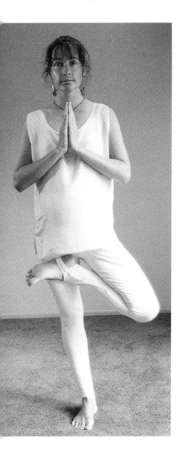 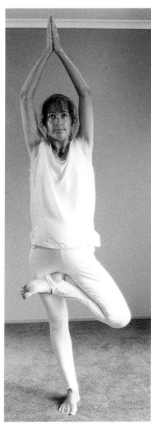

This is known as the Dynamic Tree. From this position a full stretch is felt in the sides of your body and throughout your spinal column. Some people find it easier to balance with

their arms above their head as it gives them a sense of being tall and steady. You might like to imagine that there is an invisible cord running from the heel of your supporting foot right through the crown of your head to beyond your fingertips, stretching your spine and holding you tall and straight.

Note: When practising the Tree do not 'sit down' into your hip, as you might have seen photos of nomadic people doing, but lift up through your leg so that the sides of your body are straight, and your body is tall and erect.

2. The Eagle
(garudasana)

This posture was named after the mythical eagle Garuda who was half man, half eagle and was said to be the vehicle for the Hindu god, Vishnu. It is also named after the eagle which is considered to be king among birds and possessor of great power and strength.

The benefits gained from practising the Eagle can be divided between your upper body and your lower body. In your upper body, a deep stretch is felt in your shoulders, upper arms, hands and fingers. Likewise a full stretch is felt across your upper back and your shoulders. This movement is very useful for removing stiffness and tension in those parts of your body. This is especially beneficial for people with arthritis or rheumatism.

In your lower body your hips, thighs, knees and ankles are deeply toned, improving circulation and nerve tone to your lower limbs. It is an excellent posture to do if leg cramps and sciatica are a problem. It also plays an important role in relieving varicose veins.

With your upper legs tightly crossed and your body bent slightly forward, your pelvic floor and upper body are nourished with a replenished blood supply. The further forward you bend and feel a deep 'squeezing' into your pelvic area, the more intense will be the benefits. However, I do not recommended you hold your body forward and squeeze tightly after the second or third month of pregnancy but stand with your body upright instead. The benefits will still be felt in your upper and lower body in this upright position, without applying too much pressure to your pelvic area.

1. Begin by standing with your body straight and your focus on a stationary object.

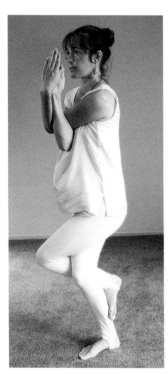

2. Extend your arms out in front of you at shoulder height. Cross your right arm over your left arm above your elbows or as high up your arms as possible. In this position you will feel a deep stretch across your back and your shoulders.

3. Bend your elbows and fold your arms inwards with your palms facing each other. Draw your arms in towards your body joining your fingers and palms. Hold your hands in front of your face and your arms close to your body.

4. Bend your knees slightly as you cross your right leg over your left leg, so they are tightly squeezed at the upper thigh. Tuck your right foot behind your left calf muscle. Lean your body a little forward over your legs,

'sitting down' into the position and squeezing deeply into your pelvic area. Hold the final posture and relax your breathing for up to nine breaths.

5. When you are ready, come out of the posture. Breathe in while unfolding your arms and legs. Shake your legs and arms before repeating the exercise with your left arm and left leg crossing over your right, reversing all the movements and completing the posture on both sides. It is important to take into account how you feel while practising the Eagle. Adjust your position to suit your size and stage of pregnancy.

3. The 'T' balance
(eka padasana)

This posture, which is also known as the Single Foot posture, has been modified for pregnancy. It is an energetic posture where the body is stretched and strengthened. It can be practised while standing unaided, but for pregnancy it is preferable to support yourself by resting your hands on the back of a chair or another suitable object of the correct height. As your body is in a horizontal position the weight of your abdomen is redistributed away from your pelvic region, which can be very useful if you are carrying low or have a lot of pressure and heaviness in your pelvis.

When practising this posture, be sure that your body is centrally balanced on the supporting leg as you reach forward with your arms. At the same time, stretch out your raised leg. As this is done you will feel a full stretch along your arms to your fingertips and from your hip through to your toes. This two-way action will keep you centrally balanced and supply a complete stretch in your arms, your back and the extended leg. In the final position you will resemble the letter 'T'.

The supporting leg is toned and strengthened in this balance. For the best results hold the leg straight. This posture builds strength and endurance but some people might find it quite strenuous to do. It is therefore important to be fully aware of how you are feeling and only hold the final position while you remain comfortable and relaxed. There is nothing to be gained if you are feeling tense or experiencing difficulty while holding the posture. If you feel this posture is completely unsuitable, practise one of the other balances instead.

1. Stand with your body straight and your feet together. Breathe in to prepare your focus and become centred.

2. Breathe out as you lift your

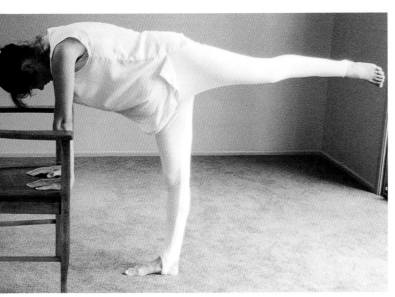

right leg and at the same time lower your body into the horizontal position. Stretch your arms out in front of you to rest on a suitable support.

3. Hold your head relaxed, either looking ahead of you or down at the floor. When your extended leg, back and arms are in a straight line you are in the final position. Hold the posture for a short time to begin with. If you find the posture to your liking then extend

the time up to five breaths. Even though this is a modified form of the 'T' posture, I feel that five breaths is long enough.

4. Inhale as you return to the standing position. Rest your legs before repeating the posture by raising your left leg.

4. The Crane
(bakasana)

The Crane is a graceful yoga *asana* that can be safely practised throughout your pregnancy, preferably in the modified form. The traditional Crane is practised with your hands resting on the floor, but I do not recommend this unless you have been practising yoga before your pregnancy and are able to do this posture easily.

Suitable alternatives would be to place your hands on the seat or back of a steady chair, on a step, or even resting on a window ledge. It is your choice where you place your hands and it depends on your degree of flexibility and where you feel the most relaxed and comfortable.

The Crane is an excellent posture for toning and strengthening your leg muscles, especially your thighs and hips. Greater strength and improved circulation will be gained in both the extended leg and the supporting leg. The supporting leg is held straight, which stretches your hamstrings and thigh muscles. Relaxation is encouraged in your lower back.

Your head is down which improves circulation to your brain, aiding concentration and mental

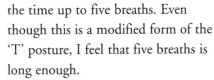

alertness and relieving fatigue. This is because your brain receives a greater blood supply when your head is down and the effects of gravity are reversed. If you find yourself getting tired after lunch around 2 or 3 p.m., you will find all the head down yoga postures especially beneficial. Your eyes and the muscles around your eyes are kept healthy and your facial muscles and the nerves supplying your facial tissues are replenished. The head down postures also help to improve memory, relieve sinus congestion and headaches.

Note: If you have blood pressure problems, ask your doctor's advice before proceeding with any head down postures

1. Begin by standing with your body straight and relaxed. Rest your hands on a suitable object for support.

2. Breathe in to prepare and focus. Then, while breathing out, bend over from your waist. The crown of your head should be facing the floor.

3. Raise your right leg as high as possible without bending your knee.

Your left leg is held straight but not tight.

4. Be sure that your body is completely relaxed and free of any discomfort or strain, breath quietly while holding the posture.

5. When you are ready to come out of the posture, breathe in to lower your leg and slowly return to a standing position. Always stand up slowly to prevent light-headedness, especially if you have high or low blood pressure.

6. Repeat the posture with your left leg raised.

5. The Dancer
(natarajasana)

Natarajasana is one of the names given to the Hindu God, Shiva, who was Lord of the Dance. This posture is dedicated to him and is sometimes called Lord Shiva's pose. In India there are many fine sculptures dedicated to this aspect of Shiva, showing figures in positions of great poise. It is an extremely graceful and beautiful posture and these qualities are passed on to all

78

The complete book of
yoga and meditation
for pregnancy

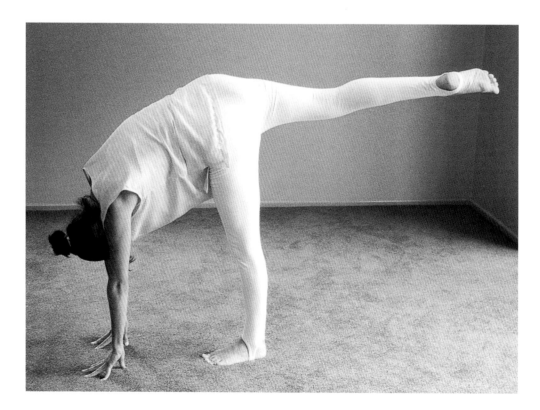

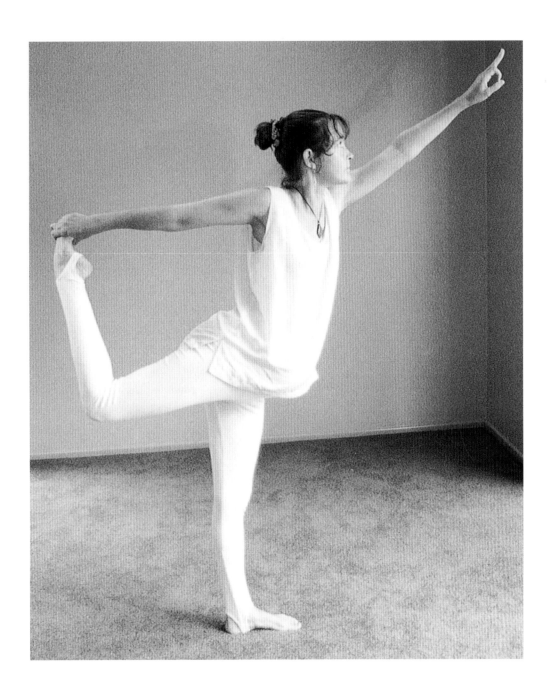

who practise it.

Lord Shiva's pose brings balance and harmony to your nervous system therefore enhancing calmness and stability in your mind and body. When this posture is practised regularly, concentration is improved so your mind becomes clearer and more alert. Like the previous postures, the supporting leg is strengthened and toned and the elevated leg is stretched and extended. This posture also enables stamina and endurance to be developed. Your chest is expanded and opened as your leg is lifted and drawn away from your body, alleviating tightness or tension from your chest and shoulders. At the same time your back is arched bringing more flexibility and suppleness to your back muscles, and tension is relieved from your middle back, hips and buttocks.

The Dancer is one of the few postures, suitable for pregnancy, where your abdominal muscles are gently stretched.

1. Stand with your body relaxed and focus on a stationary object at eye height.

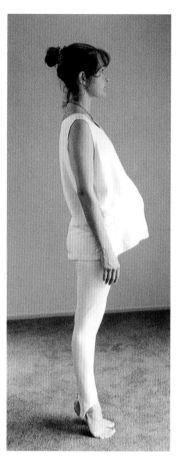

2. Take hold of the toes of your right foot with your right hand.

3. Extend your leg out behind you, lifting your leg up from

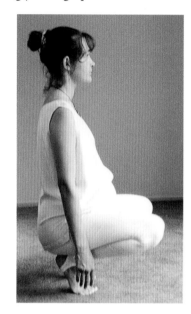

Above:
Tip toes
Right:
Squat

your hip as high as you are able to. Extend your arm back from your shoulder and stretch through your thigh and hip. In this position your leg is lifted up as well as out and away from your body. Hold your body straight in the final position.

4. Keep your shoulders relaxed and lift your left arm to eye height with your thumb and first finger joined in chin mudra. Gaze beyond your extended hand to a stationary point of focus. Relax your breathing and hold the final position for up to nine breaths. As this is a strenuous posture, you might feel that four or five breaths is ample time to hold the final position.

5. Lower your leg when you have completed your breathing and repeat the posture with your left leg raised.

Note: If you need extra support to balance while doing this posture, stand facing a wall with your fingertips in easy reach of the wall. As your

confidence grows you can move further away from the wall and only rely on it if you lose your balance.

6. Tip toes to squat

This exercise is a combination of balancing on your toes and coming into a knees-together, deep squat. It takes a little more concentrated effort as you are not standing still but are moving from a standing position to a deep squatting position. It is included here with the balancing postures because concentration, leg strength and balancing skills are needed.

As you move from the tip toe balance into the squatting position, your calf muscles and thighs are toned and strengthened. This is a very good practice for people with weak backs as it encourages the use of your thighs rather than your back. Using your leg muscles is a much better way to pick something up from the floor, rather than bending over from your waist as most people do. Your feet and toes are worked and flexibility is gained in your knees and your hips.

1. Stand with your feet together and your body straight.

2. Breathe in as you rise up onto your toes then breathe out as you move into a deep squat, keeping your back straight and your knees together for the whole exercise. When you first practise this exercise you can rest your hands on the back of a chair for support. Later on, you can rest your hands beside your body.

Repeat this exercise up to six times, being aware not to strain or become exhausted. When you have completed the desired number of squats, gently shake your legs and rotate your feet.

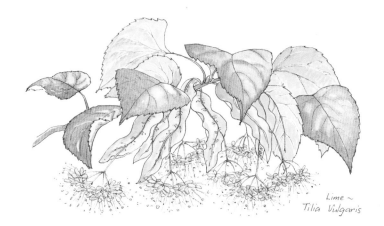

Lime ~
Tilia Vulgaris

Standing

Standing

Standing

T he standing yoga postures I
have recommended are ideal
to practise throughout your
pregnancy. They are gentle and easy
to do and they stretch and tone your
whole body. They are best practised
after the warming up exercises to give
a balanced yoga program. Choose a
few exercises and postures from that
chapter before selecting a few others
from this one.

1. The Heavenly Stretch
(tadasana)

This lovely posture will stretch
deeply yet gently throughout your
whole spinal column giving you the
feeling of being tall, balanced and
centred. Your abdominal and intestinal
areas are stretched and toned and your
abdominal muscles are also developed.

The Heavenly Stretch helps
remove any congestion in the nerves
and muscles of your spine, giving health
and suppleness throughout your back.

Your feet and lower leg muscles are
strengthened and your feet receive extra
benefits from balancing on your toes.
However, if you are unsteady on your
toes it is quite acceptable to practise this
posture without coming up onto your
toes. Stand on flat feet, instead.

The Heavenly Stretch is an
excellent posture to do if you find
constipation a problem during
pregnancy. Before breakfast drink three
of four glasses of warm water with a
squeeze of lemon juice and then practise
the Heavenly Stretch and the Tree
Blowing in the Wind posture. This will
often stimulate your liver and intestines
enough to promote a normal bowel
movement. It is a wonderfully natural
way to restore normal function to your
bowel without the need for laxatives.

1. Stand with your feet together
or a little apart. Join your hands
together in front of you with your
palms facing upwards and your
shoulders relaxed.

81

Asana
Balalncing

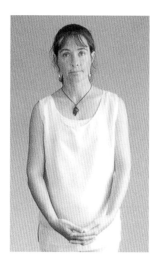

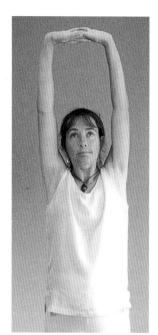

2. Breathe in as you raise your arms above your head, rising up onto your toes and balancing, with your palms facing the ceiling. Keep your shoulders relaxed and hold your breath briefly while you balance on your toes. It is not recommended that you hold your breath for lengthy periods during pregnancy but this short pause is quite acceptable and will not cause you any distress.

3. Breathe out as you lower your arms and heels and return to the standing position. Repeat this up to nine times. It is helpful to focus on a stationary object before commencing the practice because it requires balance and steadiness to stretch while on your toes.

2. The Tree Blowing in the Wind (*tiryaka tadasana*)

This posture is a variation of the Heavenly Stretch with the addition of a swaying movement, like a tree blowing in the wind. If you feel you are unable to balance on your toes and sway from side to side, remain on flat feet and complete the posture that way. Before you begin this exercise, focus on a stationary object to help keep you balanced.

As with all balancing postures, the Tree Blowing in the Wind will help improve your concentration. In addition, your spinal column will be stretched lengthwise and sideways, keeping you supple and tension free through your back. As your body sways, your digestive system is gently squeezed

and massaged and your waist is toned. When you lift onto your toes, your lower leg and feet muscles are exercised.

1. Breathe in as you raise your arms above your head and rise up onto your toes.

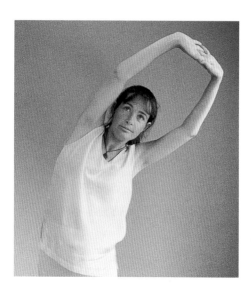

2. Breathe naturally while holding the stretch and sway, as slowly as possible, to the right and then to the left. Repeat this three times to each side before coming back to the centre.

3. Breathe in and stretch tall through your body then breathe out as you lower your arms and return your heels to the floor. Lightly shake your feet and legs after completion.

3. Arm Stretching

Both of these movements are practised in a similar way, but the manner in which they are done is quite different and the feeling in your arms and body is unrelated from the first exercise to the second.

The first movement emphasises stretching strongly and completely from your shoulders to your fingertips and feeling a deep, full stretch in the corresponding parts of your body. In the second exercise your arms literally float up and down.

Although the second exercise is

82

The complete book of
yoga and meditation
for pregnancy

not a traditional yoga posture, it will bring your awareness to a soft, light energy in your being. Your arms seem to lift gracefully – as if by themselves – and float down as light as feathers. It is wonderful to notice the different sensations of these exercises as you consciously create strength or softness by the degree of energy you apply.

Arm stretching with a deep stretch

1. Stand with your feet slightly apart and your arms relaxed beside your body.

2. Breathe in, then slowly raise your right arm out to the side and up above your head. Stretching strongly through your arm and the side of your

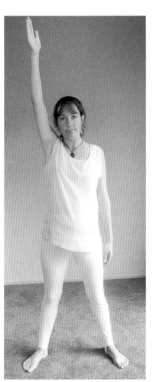
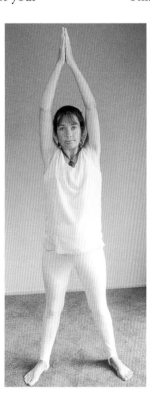

body to your hand and fingertips. Remember to keep your shoulder relaxed when your arm is above your head.

3. Breathe out and lower your arm. Reach out from your shoulder and stretch deeply into your hand and fingers as your arm drops. Repeat this three times with your right arm and

then three times with your left arm. Shake your arms lightly when you have completed the stretch.

4. Raise both arms together while breathing in. Join the palms of your hands above your head and keep your shoulders relaxed.

5. Breathe out as you lower your arms while stretching and extending them out to the sides. Repeat this movement three times. Your arms will feel warm after this exercise, which indicates the benefits you are receiving. Shake your arms lightly after completion.

Arms floating

This exercise has a very calming and relaxing effect on your body and mind. There is no need to do it with any specific breath awareness but rather to breathe quietly as your arms move softly up and down.

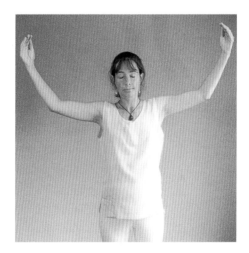

Gently allow both arms to lift out to the sides and above your head – almost by themselves – in a soft, floating movement. Think of your arms as weightless like feathers. When you are ready, allow your arms to float down slowly – palms facing upwards – like your world is now in slow motion. This movement can take as long as you like, maybe breathing two or three times while lifting your arms and a similar number to lower them. You will notice how completely different this exercise feels from the previous exercise.

Repeat this three times or more if desired. It is advantageous to do this exercise with your

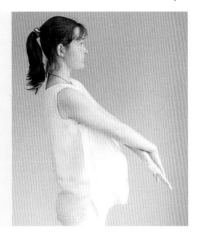

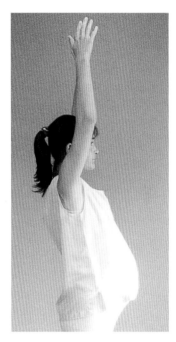

eyes closed and to be completely mindful of how you are feeling.

4. Chest Expansion with Deep Breathing
(hasta utthanasana)

There are many important benefits to be gained from practising this posture, particularly for your chest, arms, shoulders and upper back. You will notice that when your arms are behind you your chest expands fully, which assists in efficient deep breathing. Many people hold tension in the muscles of their chest, upper back and shoulders and this exercise works on easing that tightness.

When this exercise is practised regularly, all the muscles of your upper body are massaged. Your arms are stretched and toned and your shoulder joints are kept flexible, mobile and free. Circulation is improved to your lungs and upper body. This is also a very suitable remedy for round shoulders,

poor posture and inefficient breathing. People who have respiratory disorders such as asthma or emphysema are encouraged to practise this exercise as often as possible. The Chest Expansion is one of the few postures to work deeply and thoroughly into your upper body. I recommend practising it in the morning to loosen your body and at the end of the day to relieve any tightness that may have built up during the day.

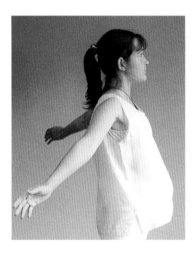

1. Stand with your body straight and your shoulders and arms relaxed. Place your right hand in front of your left hand. Keep your arms straight and relaxed.

2. Breathe in as you raise your arms up in front of your body, finishing the inhalation when your arms are above your head.

3. Breathe out as you take your arms back as far as possible while expanding your chest. When your chest is fully opened you will feel your shoulder blades and the muscles of your upper back squeeze together. Repeat this five or more times, being aware to inhale and exhale deeply with your arm movements.

84

The complete book of
yoga and meditation
for pregnancy

5. Chest Expansion with a Hamstring Stretch

In this posture your upper body will receive the same benefits as for the previous exercise. Also, your hamstrings and thigh muscles are stretched when you move your body forward.

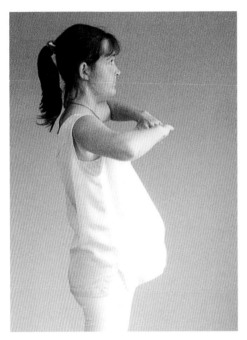

1. Stand with your feet facing the front, about a metre apart. Bend your arms and touch your fingertips together in front of the centre of your chest. Keep your palms facing down and your shoulders relaxed.

2. Breathe in and extend your arms out to the front and then to the sides until you are fully expanding your chest.

3. Breathe out as you bend forward from the hips and take your arms back as far as possible. You will feel a stretch in the backs of your legs.

4. Breathe in as you stand up again then breathe out as you reverse the arm movement and return your hands to the centre of your chest. Repeat this exercise five times or more if desired.

6. Waist Rotation and Spinal Twist
(kati chakrasana)

When it is practised regularly your spine is loosened in preparation for all other forward bending, sideways bending and spinal twist postures. It also helps with stiffness and tightness in

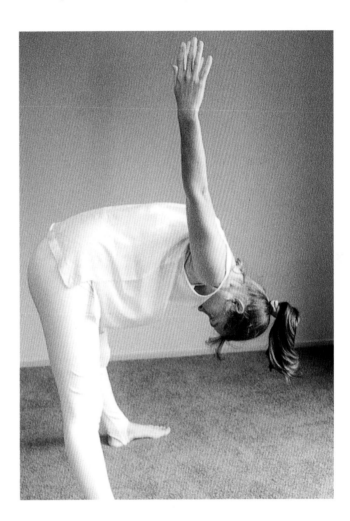

your shoulders and back and tones your waist area. This exercise could easily be included in the chapter 'Warming Up', especially before practising postures where the spine is required to bend or twist.

1. Stand with your feet about a metre apart. Breathe in while raising your arms to the sides at shoulder height.

2. Breathe out and swing your body as far to the right as possible, wrapping your arms around your body and looking over your right shoulder.

Chest Expansion with a Hamstring Stretch

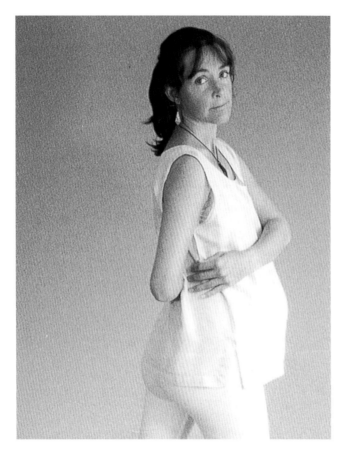

3. Breathe in and return to the centre front with your arms extended to the side.

4. Breathe out and turn your body to the left, looking over your left shoulder.

Repeat this up to nine times each side remembering to breathe with the movements.

Caution: If you have a history of high or low blood pressure or tend to become dizzy and light-headed after having your head down, either ask your doctor for advice or, if you still want to do the head down postures, proceed slowly and return to a standing position very, very gradually. For example, take two or three breaths to return to the upright position to prevent any light-headedness or dizziness.

The benefits for all head down postures.

1. Sinus congestion can be relieved and is often completely removed because your nose and nasal passages receive extra blood flow.

2. Often these postures will help to alleviate headaches, as the weight of your head will stretch your neck muscles, relieving tension and tightness in this area.

3. Circulation to your head and especially your brain is definitely improved. Memory and concentration are also enhanced. Mental fatigue is removed and if these postures are practised around 2 or 3 p.m. (when gravity is at its greatest), you will notice an increased clarity and general alertness for the remainder of the day.

4. Blood flow to the pituitary gland – the master gland of the endocrine system – is improved, helping to enhance the function of the whole hormonal system.

5. The nervous system is balanced when the head is down, which encourages mental and emotional stress to be relieved, and more harmony to be experienced throughout the body and the mind. You will also appreciate an improvement in physical wellbeing.

6. Your hair and scalp are kept healthy and problems such as dandruff can be rectified with regular practice, due to the increased blood supply to your head.

7. As the blood flow to your face is greatly improved, your eyes and the muscles around your eyes will benefit. This will help prevent wrinkles and ease facial tension.

86

The complete book of
yoga and meditation
for pregnancy

7. The Pose of Two Angles
(dwi konasana)

This is a good posture for removing tightness from your shoulders and upper back. Often, the muscles between your shoulder blades become rigid due to stress or poor posture, and extending your arms up behind your back is an effective way of loosening these muscles. *Dwi konasana* is also one of the few exercises to work effectively into the muscles of your upper arms.

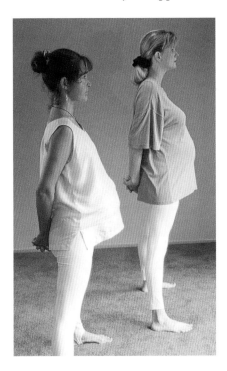

When people first attempt this posture it is quite common for their arms not to extend very far away from their back. With practice however, your arms, shoulders and chest will free up enough for you to notice a considerable difference in the extension you are achieving. This exercise expands your chest muscles in a similar way to *hasta uttanasana*, which is excellent for establishing more efficient breathing.

1. Stand with your feet facing the front about a metre apart. Join your hands together behind your back and relax your shoulders.

2. Breathe in to prepare and as you breathe out bend your body forward at the hips. The top of your head should be facing the floor. Extend your arms away from your body as far as is comfortable. Hold this posture as you breathe in a relaxed and natural manner.

3. Breathe in as you return slowly to a standing position. This exercise can be repeated up to three times.

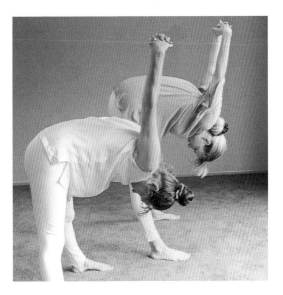

8. The Triangle Side Bend
(trikonasana)

Trikonasana, the full side bending posture is a significant yoga practice with many benefits for the pregnant woman. It is completely safe to practise during pregnancy but if you find the full side bend uncomfortable, particularly in the last few weeks, it can be varied and modified to suit your individual needs and level of flexibility. Some people are very supple in all the sideways bending positions but others will find the spinal twists or the forward bends easier to do. The important point to remember is how the posture is practised; with the emphasis on full body, mind and breath awareness rather than how far you have extended.

The Side Bend is often considered quite a dynamic posture and it is necessary to be quite precise in the way your body is positioned so as to achieve all the benefits and remain balanced. There is a tendency to bend slightly forward instead of to the side, so it is a good idea to practise this posture with your back against a wall as a way of keeping your body square to the front. The ideal position of the final posture is to have your right ear, right shoulder and right knee in line, so that your left shoulder does not come forward. When it is practised in this way, the degree of sideways movement will seem less but the final posture will be more exact.

This is a most enjoyable stretch to practise during pregnancy and it provides a number of wonderful benefits. The sides of your body receive either a full stretch or a deep squeeze. For example, as your body is flexed to the right, your liver and the right side of your bowel are massaged, which assists in establishing optimum function. This is important if there is a problem with a sluggish liver, minor digestive disorders and constipation. Alternatively, as your body is leant to the left, your spleen and pancreas are benefited and the left side of your bowel is massaged. Also, your spinal column is stretched sideways increasing flexibility and your lower back, hip and inner thigh muscles are stretched.

Trikonasana is a good example of a 'passive yet dynamic' yoga posture, in that it is enjoyable and gentle, but at the same time provides dynamic benefits to many parts of your body. I recommend this posture be included in all your yoga programs.

1. Stand with your feet about a metre apart with your left foot facing to the front and your right foot turned out to the right. Keep your hips and shoulders in line and square to the front.

2. Breathe in and raise your arms to the sides at shoulder height, keeping your shoulders relaxed. Feel the energy flowing from your shoulders to your fingertips as you stretch your arms.

3. Breathe out and bend your body to the right. Rest your right hand

The complete book of
**yoga and meditation
for pregnancy**

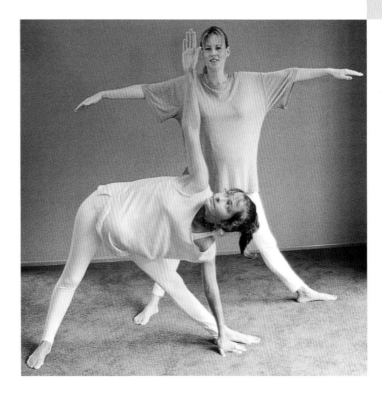

on your right leg. Raise your left arm to a vertical position and gaze at your left thumb. Adjust the position where your hand rests on your leg so as to modify the depth of the side bend to best suit your level of flexibility. Remain relaxed while holding the final posture and breathe quietly for up to nine breaths.

When you first practise the side bend, remain in the final posture for only two or three breaths so as to adjust to the tilted position. When you are ready, increase the length of time you remain in the posture. If you have neck problems and are unable to easily look at your extended hand, either look straight ahead or look down at your foot.

4. Breathe in as you return to the standing position then lower your arms while breathing out. Repeat the side bend to the left, reversing all the procedures.

Note: It is also acceptable to have your knee bent instead of straight, especially if you are finding the inner thigh stretch too strong. For example, when you are bending to the right, your right knee can be slightly bent. The benefits to the side of your body are exactly the same, the only difference is to your inner thigh area.

9. The Hero

The Hero is another of the triangle postures, and like *trikonasana*, is a passive but dynamic exercise. It looks fairly simple and straightforward but care needs to be taken not to hold the final posture for too long, as fatigue will result from overexertion. These strong, static yoga postures are beneficial for building strength, tenacity and endurance in the physical body. They also influence mental and emotional stamina and help to develop the much sought after inner strength which is so

important during labour.

Specifically, the Hero will strengthen your thigh, inner thigh and calf muscles while bringing tone to your whole body. Because your arms are held up and stretched they will become stronger the more the posture is practised. The Hero will also give you a feeling of balance and steadiness.

1. Stand with your feet at least a metre apart. Turn your right foot to the right and your left foot to the front. Face your body square to the front and turn your head to the right. For maximum benefits, make sure your feet

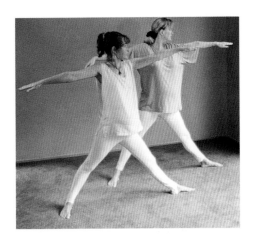

are wide enough apart for you to move deeply into the posture.

2. Inhale as you raise your arms to the sides, looking out along your right arm. Then exhale while bending your right leg, keeping your lower leg

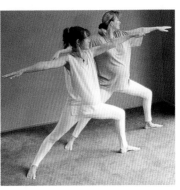

straight upright from your ankle to your knee. You will feel a deep stretch up the inside of your left leg and strength in your right thigh. Relax your shoulders. Hold this posture for up to nine breaths, however if you are finding it strenuous only hold the final posture for two or three breaths until your strength increases.

3. Inhale as you straighten your right leg, then exhale as you lower your arms. Repeat this to your left, reversing all the above directions.

4. Shake your legs lightly when you have completed the posture.

10. The Warrior
(virabhadrasana)

The Warrior is another of the triangle postures. It gives wonderful benefits to your legs and increases your strength and endurance. I have modified the original posture only slightly for the purposes of pregnancy because I feel the full posture – where your arms are up above your head – is generally too strenuous for pregnant women.

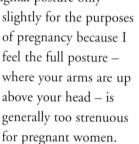

1. Stand with your feet about a meter apart and with your toes facing forward. Turn your body to the

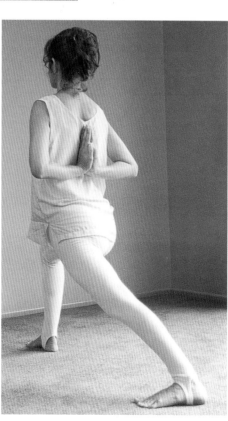

right. Your right foot faces in the same direction as the front of your body and your left foot is turned slightly inwards. In this posture you will feel a stretch in your left calf muscle and your ankle. Join your hands in the prayer position at the centre of your chest, or at the centre of your back.

2. Breathe in to prepare then, as you breathe out, bend your right leg and lunge as deeply as you can while remaining comfortable. Keep your right lower leg vertical from the ankle to the knee and your left leg straight.

3. Hold the posture and breathe quietly for up to nine breaths. If you find this a particularly strenuous posture, only hold it for a short time.

4. Breathe in as you return to the standing position, breathe out and relax.

5. Turn your body to the left and repeat the Warrior on that side.

11. The Intense Forward Stretch
(parsvottanasana)

The word 'intense' is used here to describe the stretch in the hamstrings rather than to discourage you from attempting this posture. Although it is a very strong stretch it is not considered an advanced yoga posture and it is an ideal exercise to practise during pregnancy.

Note: As this is a head down posture there is a caution for people who have high or low blood pressure, details of which can be found outlined previously. However, if those guidelines are followed there is no reason why this posture cannot be practised.

All benefits for the head down postures apply for this posture, as well as those gained from the full arm extension. This posture will extend your spine, encouraging suppleness throughout your back. Also, your hips, the muscles behind your knees and your

90

The complete book of
yoga and meditation
for pregnancy

hamstrings are stretched and toned. Do not force your body beyond what is a comfortable forward bend because that will only create more stiffness the next day. Your abdomen and pelvis are gently massaged by the posture and circulation is improved to those parts of your body. Even at full term, this is a comfortable and acceptable posture for you to practise.

1. Prepare for this posture by standing with your feet facing the front about a metre apart. Join your hands behind your back either in the prayer position or with your arms relaxed and fingers entwined, and relax your shoulders.

2. Turn your body and your right foot to the right. Turn your left foot slightly inwards. When you turn your body to the right you will be square over your right leg and you will feel a definite stretch in your calf muscles. I suggest that your right foot be moved even further out to the right, to make it easier to maintain balance when bending forward. This is a slight modification from the original posture but I feel it is quite an acceptable one for pregnancy. When you are ready and in position, breathe in to prepare.

3. Breathe out and extend your body over your right leg, bringing your head down towards your knee. Stretch your arms up and away from your body. The top of your head should be facing the floor and your neck muscles relaxed. I have noticed that many people are inclined to hold the head slightly up in the head down postures, causing tension

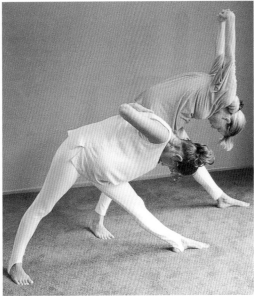

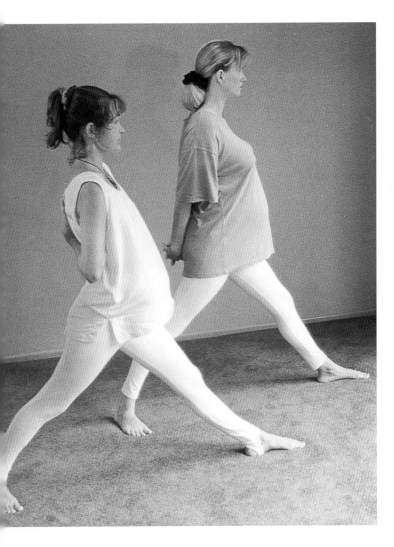

in the neck and the upper back. This also prevents efficient circulation flowing to your face and your brain, which is one of the main reasons why these postures are so encouraged.

4. Hold the posture for three breaths before inhaling as you return to the standing position.

5. Repeat the movement once more over your right leg.

6. Turn your body back to the front and then to the left. Follow all the instructions to repeat the posture over your left leg. When you have completed the posture, release your hands and shake them lightly.

12. The Forward Bend
(pada hastasana)

During pregnancy, it is advised to practise this posture with your feet slightly apart and to follow all the usual precautions and guidelines for head down postures. If you are having back problems it would be better to practise the Wide-A Leg Stretch instead of this one, due to the extent of the stretch on your back muscles.

A friend of mine is a physiotherapist and he recommends for people with a weak or damaged lower back to always return to the standing position with their legs slightly bent to prevent extra strain on the back muscles.

A modification for later in pregnancy, is to stand with your feet apart and hold onto the back of a chair or a stable piece of furniture at an appropriate height, and bend over from that position. You will still notice all the benefits of the Forward Bend but with a little extra support and slightly less stretch on your leg muscles.

This posture has a very beneficial effect on your digestive system because of the position of the body in the

forward bend. It will assist in more efficient digestion and help to remove such problems as constipation, flatulence and acidity. At the same time your pelvis and abdomen are gently massaged. Your spinal column is stretched and your central nerves are toned. Your hamstrings and thigh muscles are stretched, and a full extension is felt throughout your legs. As with all the standing postures, it is important not to overextend or cause strain in your body.

1. Stand with your feet half a metre apart and bring your awareness to your whole body.

2. Breathe in deeply to prepare. Breathe out as you bend your body forward from the waist. The top of your head should be facing the floor allowing your neck and shoulder muscles to remain relaxed. When you first practise this posture you might notice a fullness in your face but with practise this sensation will pass and you will feel very relaxed. Relax your arms and let them

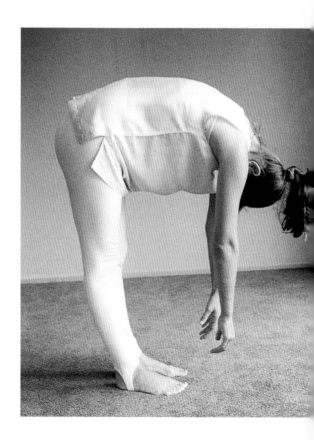

92

The complete book of
yoga and meditation
for pregnancy

fall freely from your shoulders. Depending on your level of flexibility, your hands can rest either on your legs or on your feet. Do not push yourself further into this final posture than is comfortable. Remain relaxed at all times. Hold the posture for up to nine breaths.

3. Breathe in as you slowly straighten your spine and return to the standing position. Always return to the upright position as slowly as possible to prevent dizziness. If need be, take two breaths when returning to the standing position.

13. Wide-A Leg Stretch
(prasavita padottanasana)

Before practising this stretch, I suggest you first check whether you are able to comfortably and easily reach the floor with your hands, without bending your knees or straining your inner thigh muscles. The Wide-A Leg Stretch is a strong posture which gives a deep stretch to your inner thigh muscles. It is very important not to extend so far that you feel pain rather than a stretch. To achieve all the true benefits of yoga, the focus needs to be on stretch and extension, never on pain.

When you first attempt this posture, begin by resting your hands on the back of a chair, or some other suitable object, instead of reaching for the floor. In this way you can gradually ease into the full posture without the risk of straining your body. With practise, your inner thigh muscles will become more flexible and you will be able to reach the floor with your hands.

Your inner thigh muscles and the muscles and ligaments of your pelvic floor are toned deeply by this wide leg stretch. It is extremely important to prepare these muscles for childbirth as they need to be strong and supple

during and after the birth.

Although this stretch is not a posture where your back is extended fully, it will still help to stretch the muscles of your back and neck. Your lower back is opened and lightly stretched. I have found many pregnant women really enjoy this posture especially if sciatica is a problem. If you have a back problem, it is recommended that you do not bend forward with your feet together but instead stretch forward with your legs wide apart as in this exercise.

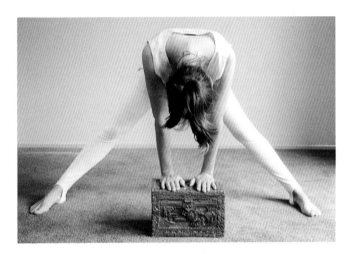

This posture is also recommended for later in pregnancy when many women experience considerable strain in the groin area due to the weight of the pregnancy. This posture seems to move the weight away from that area. All benefits apply to this posture as detailed for other head down positions.

1. Begin by standing with your feet about a metre apart and slowly separate your legs to a distance that is comfortable for you. When your legs are in position, lower your hands either to a chair, a step, or to the floor and drop your head down so that the top of your head is facing the floor. If your feet are inclined to slip, one foot can be placed against a wall for support, and if you are on carpet take your socks off. Never

have your legs so wide in this posture that you are finding it more of a strain than simply a stretch. It is very important to always remember to take responsibility for how you are feeling in a posture, and only work within your own level of flexibility and in complete comfort.

2. Hold the final posture for up to nine breaths. You will notice that the longer you remain in this posture the

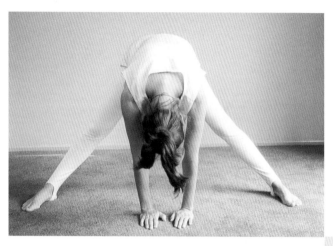

more relaxed your back and inner thigh muscles become as you breathe and move more completely into the stretch. As with all inverted postures, your mind will gradually become quiet and still.

3. Bring your feet closer together and stand up very slowly while breathing in. Shake your legs lightly when the posture is completed.

14. The Mountain
(parvatasana)

This wonderful posture has been called both the Mountain and the Dog *(adho mukha svanasana)* in traditional yoga texts and both names describe it well. More recently, it has also been called the Dolphin! This posture resembles a dog stretching and pulling its body strongly towards its back legs. It also looks like a mountain peak, your buttocks and lower back being the summit, your arms and your head

resembling one side of the mountain and your legs and feet the other side.

It is probably one of the best postures for extending your hamstrings and thigh muscles and for deeply stretching your back. However, care needs to be taken as it can be quite an intense posture and may not be enjoyed by everyone. For that reason, it is important to ease slowly into the full stretch where your heels are on the floor or quite close to the floor and to spend time in the final posture as well as resting away from it.

I have found that many people are tight in the hamstrings and thigh muscles and when first attempting this posture they comment on how strong the stretch is and how tight their hamstrings and muscles really are. Nevertheless, do not be discouraged because with time this can become an enjoyable posture and the benefits definitely outweigh any beginner's discomfort. During pregnancy, I have found the majority of women enjoy this posture but if you find it's not suitable, practise one of the other inverted postures instead.

The Mountain has many benefits, including all those mentioned for the inverted postures where your head is lower than your heart. Other benefits include:

- Tightness and tension are released from your hamstrings, thigh and calf muscles, and your ankles become more flexible.
- Your spinal column is stretched and your spinal nerves are toned which has a nourishing and rejuvenating effect on your whole body.
- The muscles of your back are extended fully, keeping your back flexible and strong.
- Tired and aching legs are relieved, muscle cramps are often removed

The complete book of
yoga and meditation
for pregnancy

and circulation to your legs is generally improved.

- It is one of the postures recommended for relieving backache or sciatica pain, often common problems during pregnancy.
- Circulation to your arms and hands is increased and the Mountain is very beneficial during the later stages of pregnancy, especially if you have numbness or a fluid build-up in your hands.
- The Mountain is considered a safe posture to do if you have high or low blood pressure when it is approached in a sensible manner, keeping in mind to always return to the standing position slowly. If you are unsure, seek advice from your doctor.

A friend of mine used the Mountain to great benefit during the later part of her labour, to help slow down the contractions and to give relief from the intense pressure she was feeling in the perineum. This is detailed in the 'Birth Journeys' section of the book.

1. Rest on your hands and knees. Have your knees the same distance apart as your shoulders and your hands directly under your shoulders.

2. When you are ready, straighten your legs by lifting your hips upwards and gently ease your heels towards the floor. Hang your head in a relaxed way in between your shoulders so that the muscles of your neck remain loose and relaxed. When you are in this posture, feel as if your hips are being drawn back towards your heels. Feel the stretch in your back and spinal column. Hold the

posture for the length of time that suits you best, remembering to breathe quietly and naturally.

To gain relief from the deep stretch in the backs of your legs, lift your heels off the floor from time to time or return to your knees until you are ready to continue on with the posture. Remember not to remain in the stretch if you are feeling a lot of discomfort in your legs or fullness in your face.

3. On completion, return to your knees and then relax in the Pose of the Hare, either with your head resting on your hands or with your arms stretched out in front of you.

15. Pelvic Rocking

Although Pelvic Rocking is not a traditional yoga exercise, it has many important benefits to offer during pregnancy, and it is fun. It can be practised in a kneeling position and in an all-fours position, but many women prefer to stand with their legs apart and their knees slightly bent. It is done by slowly rotating your whole pelvic area in full circular movements, first clockwise then anticlockwise as many times as desired.

This exercise has a massaging and relaxing effect on your lower abdominal and pelvic areas, and is sometimes used during labour to free your pelvis and encourage the baby to move down through the birth canal. It is interesting to note its connection to Belly Dancing which is becoming a popular form of exercise for women, with many obvious benefits for pregnancy.

Valerian officinalis

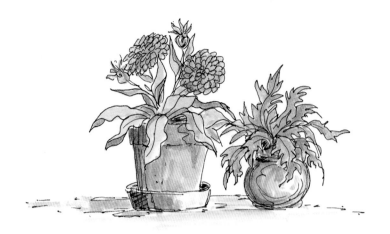

Spinal Twists

Matsyendra was one of the founders of Hatha Yoga and the Spinal Twists are known as *matsyendrasana* after him. There are a number of Spinal Twists detailed in this chapter with the specific view of pregnancy in mind. They include twists practised in a standing position, in a seated position, sitting in a chair and lying on the floor.

In advanced yoga practices there are a number of complicated variations of the Spinal Twists, which are extremely difficult to do and are only suitable for experienced yoga students. However, the postures and exercises I have recommended here range from the most simple and least demanding on your body to a slightly modified full posture that most women find very beneficial and easy to do.

I don't feel any yoga program is complete without including the Spinal Twists, as they are designed to work the central network within the body's structure, that being the spinal column and central nervous system.

The spinal column runs the length of your body from the base of your spine at your tail bone, to the top of your spine at the atlas which is located at the base of your skull. It is from your central nervous system that the nerves reach all areas of your body.

The nervous system can be divided into two separate but interconnected parts; the central nervous system consisting of the brain and spinal cord, and the peripheral nervous system which directs messages from the brain via the spinal column to other parts of the body. Many of the functions of our nervous system work independently of our direct involvement. For example, our heart will continue beating and our blood will circulate without us willing it to happen. Of course, there are other functions that require our conscious

96

The complete book of
yoga and meditation
for pregnancy

thoughts to create the desired response.

Physically and emotionally there are many reasons why the Spinal Twists are so valuable to incorporate into your yoga program, including the following:

- The way we think and feel and the way we live our lives, also has a significant bearing on the health of the nervous system. That is, our lifestyle directly effects how the body functions and the level of physical, mental and emotional health we experience in our day to day lives. The absolute health of the nervous system and to a lesser degree the suppleness of the spine, will undoubtedly influence the balance and wellbeing that is experienced in the whole body.

- Tension in your back – which is often caused by stress manifesting as tight muscles – is relieved. By gently moving your body into a Spinal Twist, you can loosen tight muscles and soothe your nerves. You will feel more relaxed as your whole nervous system is toned and supported.

- Your digestion is improved because the muscles and organs in your abdominal area are alternately compressed and stretched therefore assisting optimum function.

The Spinal Twists recommended can be modified to suit your individual needs, especially in the last weeks of pregnancy where your size might prevent you from comfortably practising one of the postures. It is important to feel as relaxed as possible when you are holding the final positions, so you can breathe and move deeply into the twist.

Movement in mind and body

It is widely accepted now that the quality of our thoughts has a direct impact on the way we feel and our standard of physical health. All our

conscious thoughts have an emotion attached to them, and these in turn make an impression on our physical bodies. If our thoughts are troubled or negative we will be feeling similar emotions which will be influencing our nervous system and ultimately our whole body. Often, if I am feeling rigid in my thoughts or if my attitude has been stubborn, my back will be stiff and uncomfortable and will have an – old' feeling about it.

The Spinal Twists will not change the way we think or our outlook on life but they will loosen an inflexible back and give us the opportunity to look at how much more care we need to take of our physical bodies and our thought processes. This will also provide the opportunity to delve into the immediate focus of our thoughts and unresolved emotions which we may be holding in the back and neck muscles. When the Spinal Twists are practised regularly, you will begin to notice a greater sense of wellbeing in your body and a more relaxed awareness of your inner self.

Yoga is a self nurturing, lifestyle improving opportunity, and I feel the more in tune and aware we become of the physical body, the more likely we are to begin understanding our thoughts and our feelings, realising how neither one is ever really separated from the other.

For all the seated Spinal Twists, follow this procedure:
(i) Breathe in to prepare and lift up through your spine.
(ii) Breathe out to complete the twist.
(iii) Breathe quietly and relax while holding the posture.
(iv) Breathe in as you return to the front.
(v) Breathe out as you release the posture.

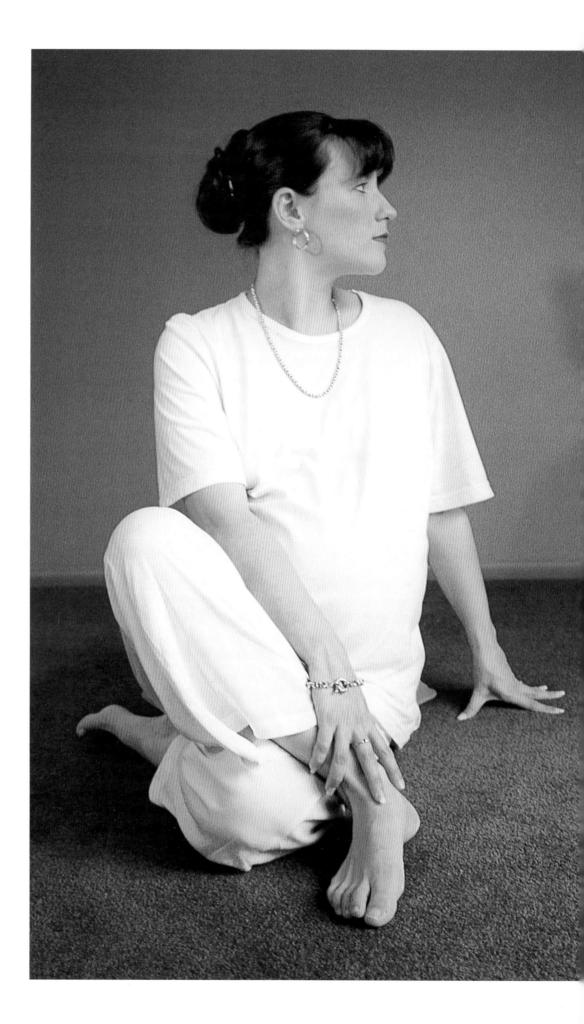

98

The complete book of
yoga and meditation
for pregnancy

Note: When practising the seated spinal twists try to feel as if you are twisting from the base of your spine rather than from the middle of your back. In other words, feel that you are lifting from the floor upwards. In this way your back is held straight before you begin turning and the full benefit of the posture will be experienced.

1. The Easy Seated Spinal Twist
(meru wakrasana)

This gentle Spinal Twist can be done with your legs in any of the three recommended positions and is an excellent way to twist the spinal column and loosen deeply throughout your back. You will feel your whole spine twisting from the base to the vertebrae of your neck.

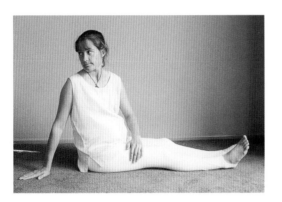

With straight legs

1. Sit on the floor with your legs in front of you and your spine straight.

2. Breathe in to prepare. Turn your body as far to the right as possible while breathing out. Look over your right shoulder and place your right hand behind your back and your left hand on the outer part of your right thigh, right knee or beside your right hip. Hold your spine straight and your shoulders relaxed while you relax into the twist. Hold the posture for up to nine breaths. The arm behind your back acts as a support for your back and also stops your body from leaning back too far.

3. Breathe in as you return to the front.

4. Change legs and repeat the twist to the left.

With one leg bent

1. Sit with your spine straight and your legs in front of you. Your right leg remains straight and your left leg is bent with your left foot placed either on the outside or the inside of your right knee.

2. Prepare as recommended in procedure (i) and turn your body to the right so that you are looking over your right shoulder. Place your right hand behind your back and your left hand on your left knee or on your right hip. When you are in a comfortable

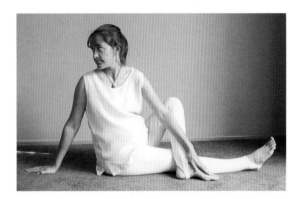

position, relax into the posture holding it for up to nine breaths.

3. Breathe in as you return to the front. Change legs to repeat the twist to the left.

With both legs bent

1. Begin with both legs to the front.

2. Bend your left leg and place your left foot alongside your right outer thigh.

3. Your right leg is folded back under you and your right foot rests beside your left hip. Your buttocks are on the floor as you sit square with your spine straight. To complete this posture

you need to have a reasonable amount of flexibility in your hips and thighs. Some women find it helpful to sit on a thin cushion when it is placed under the right hip in this case, and the left hip when the legs are reversed.

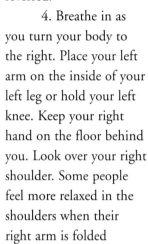

4. Breathe in as you turn your body to the right. Place your left arm on the inside of your left leg or hold your left knee. Keep your right hand on the floor behind you. Look over your right shoulder. Some people feel more relaxed in the shoulders when their right arm is folded behind their back to rest along the middle of the back.

5. Hold the final posture for up to nine breaths. Keep your awareness on relaxing your body into the twist.

6. Breathe in as you return to the front, unfolding your legs as you breathe out. Shake your legs a little when you have completed each side.

7. Repeat the twist to the other side by changing legs and turning to the left.

2. The modified Half Spinal Twist
(ardha matsyendrasana)

This *asana* has been modified for pregnancy but retains many of its original benefits. Care needs to be taken in this posture as you will find that it is a deeper twist and stretch than the previous postures, especially through the middle of your back and your abdomen. However, if you approach the modified Half Spinal Twist sensibly and in a relaxed way, it can be practised throughout your pregnancy in complete comfort.

1. Begin with your legs in the folded position described in point 3 of the previous posture. Keep your body facing forward.

2. Breathe in as you turn your body to the left. Place your left hand on

100

The complete book of
yoga and meditation
for pregnancy

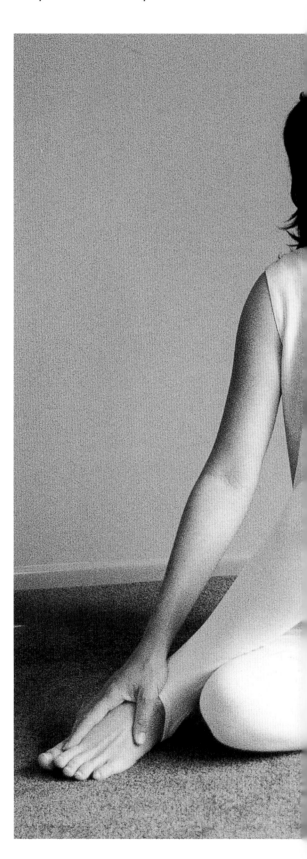

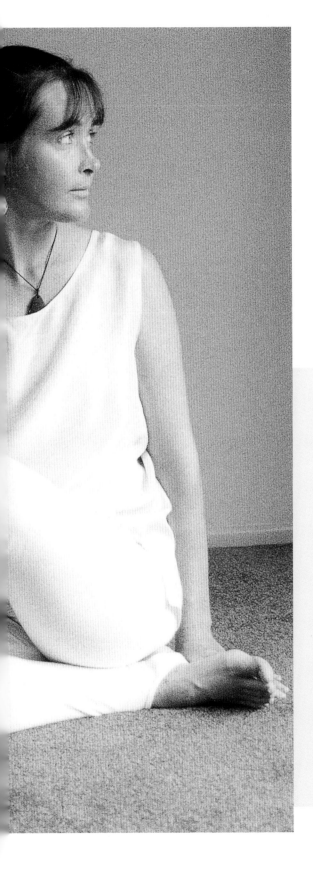

the floor behind your back. Place your right hand either on your left foot, your left knee, or on your left hip for a deeper twist. You will feel a slight twist in your abdominal area as well as in the middle of your back.

3. Breathe out as you turn your head over your left shoulder. Breathe and relax into the posture.

4. Breathe in as you turn your body to the front. Breathe out as you unfold your legs. Shake your legs lightly.

5. Repeat the twist to the other side.

It is important not to twist beyond your own level of flexibility. To improve your level of flexibility, try to practise these Spinal Twists as often as possible and you will notice a greater sense of freedom in your back. Be aware not to hold tension in your shoulders or your back when you are in the posture. Instead, breathe deeply and relax into the twist as you imagine all discomfort being dissolved and removed.

3. The Dynamic Spinal Twist
(gatyatmak meru vakrasana)

Caution: The Dynamic Spinal Twist is usually included with the seated wide leg postures, and I don't recommend you practise this exercise without first having worked into stretching and loosening your inner thigh areas. It is not advisable to do this exercise if you have a weak lower back, an injury, or if you have found the wide leg stretches are really uncomfortable. However, it is an excellent Spinal Twist and quite suitable to practise during your pregnancy, especially when it is done slowly and without straining. If you plan to include this in your yoga program, always loosen your hips and inner thigh areas first with the Hip Rotation, the Butterfly, and after practising all the other wide leg stretches.

Variation (i)

1. Begin by sitting on the floor with your legs as wide to the sides as possible and your spine straight.

2. Breathe in as you lift your arms to the sides at shoulder height.

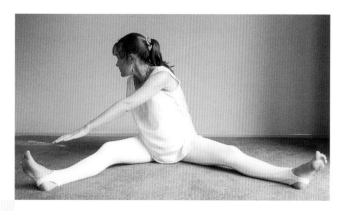

3. Breathe out as you turn your body to the right. Extend your right hand out behind you and rest your left hand on your right leg. Look over your right shoulder at your right hand. Only turn as far as you can without straining. Never overextend yourself. If possible, try to keep both legs straight.

4. Breathe in as you return to the centre front.

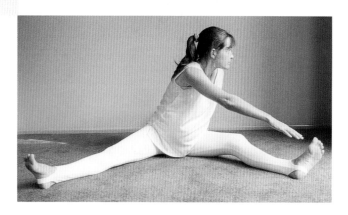

5. Breathe out as you twist your body to the left.

6. Repeat this five times to each side. Remember to breathe in as you straighten your spine each time you come to the centre front, and breath out as you twist to the left or right.

Variation (ii)

This variation is similar to the previous variation, but without the breath awareness or straightening your body each time you return to the centre front. The Dynamic Spinal Twist is loosening to your spinal column and back muscles, relieving all stiffness and tension from those areas. It is also extremely good for toning your waist and the sides of your body. This may not be an obvious concern during pregnancy but will become relevant after the birth when you will want to tone your waist again. By including this posture during pregnancy you will be able to regain your usual shape more easily.

1. Sitting in the same position as for the previous variation, simply swing your arms freely to the left and the right, allowing the weight of your body and the momentum of the movement to turn your body from side to side, slowly and easily. This is a lovely flowing movement which really frees your back and loosens your spine.

2. Repeat this exercise five times to each side. Rest by lying on your back, hug your knees into your chest and fold your arms around your knees. Gently and slowly, rock your body from side to side.

4. The Spinal Twists practised lying on your back

Note: Some women are not comfortable lying on their back later in pregnancy, so if there is any discomfort or nausea, discontinue with the practice and do one of the seated postures instead.

Both legs bent
(supta udarakarshanasana)

This exercise is good for relieving tightness in your lower back and hips.

102

The complete book of
yoga and meditation
for pregnancy

1. Lie on your back with both legs bent at the knees. Place your feet flat on the floor, hip distance apart and as close to your buttocks as possible. Spread your arms out, at shoulder level, along the floor with your palms should be facing down.

2. Breathe in to prepare. Breathe out as you lower your knees to the right and turn your head to face the left. Breathe deeply and relax. Let your knees drop as close to the floor as possible without your left shoulder lifting from the floor. If you are experiencing any discomfort in your lower back or hips,

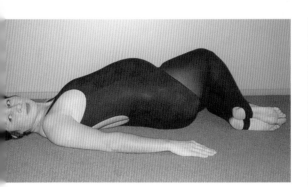

lift your knees slightly.

3. Breathe in as you bring your knees to the upright position again.

4. Breathe out as you lower your knees to the left and turn your head to face the right. Again, hold the posture as you breathe deeply and relax your back muscles and spinal column. This can be repeated up to five times each side.

5. For a dynamic variation: Repeat the exercise but, instead of holding the twist and breathing into the posture, roll from right to left as you breathe in and breathe out. This can be repeated up to five times each side. Your hands can be placed behind your head as an alternative arm position.

One leg bent and one leg straight
(shava udarakarshanasana)

I often recommend this exercise if tension in the back or stiffness in the

spine is causing a problem, repeating it both in the morning and at night. It is very interesting to notice just how much tightness can gather in the body in the course of a day.

1. Begin by lying on your back with your spine straight.

2. The left leg is straight. Bend your right leg and place your right foot either behind your left knee or on the outside of your left knee. Choose the foot position for comfort as it will not alter the effect of the posture.

3. Roll over slightly onto your left hip so that your right knee comes as

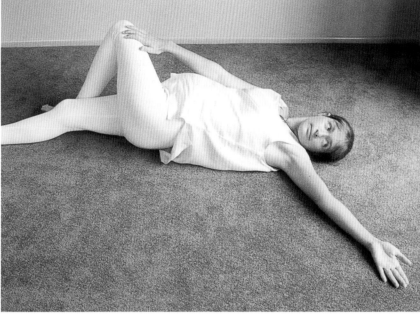

close to the floor as possible. Rest your left hand on your right knee. This will help to keep your body in the twisted position because your hand puts weight on your leg and helps to hold it in position. However, it is important not to roll over onto your hip to the point where the posture is no longer comfortable.

4. Extend your right arm along the floor at shoulder level with your palm turned upwards. Turn your head to look at your hand. Place your arm where you can easily see your hand

without straining your eyes or neck. If your right shoulder lifts off the floor, you have twisted too far to the left, so roll out of the twist to a point where your shoulder stays on the floor.

5. Be sure you are free of any tension in your right hip and lower back then ease fully into the twist.

6. Hold the final twist for up to nine breaths or longer if desired. The idea is to be as comfortable as if you were lying straight in the relaxation posture.

7. Straighten your body to come out of the twist. Then, repeat the posture to the other side by reversing all the movements.

Single leg lift with Spinal Twist

This posture will benefit your spine and back muscles, strengthen your legs and tone your abdominal muscles.

If you find this posture too strenuous, especially later in pregnancy, replace it with the *supta udarakarshanasana*, exercise (i).

1. Begin by lying on your back with your spine straight. Hold your arms out to the side at shoulder level with your palms facing down.

2. Breathe in as you slowly raise your right leg as high as you comfortably can. Keep your leg straight.

3. Breathe out as you take your right leg over your body in the direction of your left hand, as you roll over onto your left hip. Keep your shoulders on the floor, and turn your head to the right.

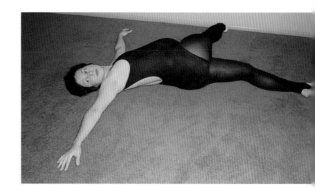

4. Breathe in as you raise your leg to the upright position.

5. Breathe out as you lower your leg to the floor.

6. Repeat this twice more with your right leg, then repeat the exercise with your left leg.

5. Spinal Twist practised in a chair

This gentle exercise is especially useful for anyone who is not comfortable either in the seated Spinal Twists or the Spinal Twists practised lying on the floor. It has similar benefits to the other exercises as it works very deeply into your back, but has been modified for comfort. Because of the simplicity of the posture, it can be done any time you are sitting in a chair and you need to relieve stiffness in your back.

1. Sit in a straight-backed chair with your spine straight, your legs uncrossed and your feet on the floor. Put a small box or a thick

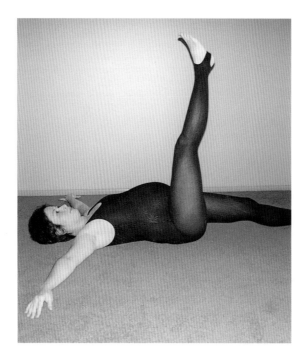

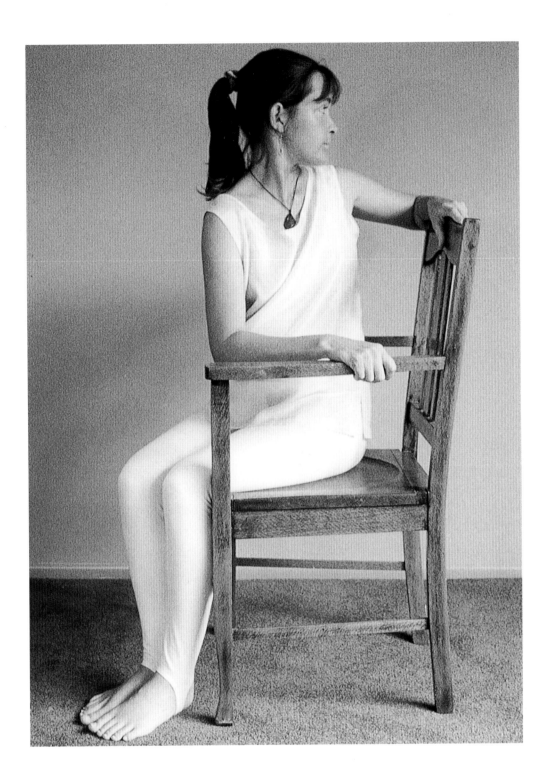

book under each foot if your feet don't reach the floor.

    2. Turn your body to the right and hold the back of the chair with your right hand and the seat with your left hand.

    3. Relax your shoulders and turn your head to look over your right shoulder. Hold the twist as you breathe quietly.

    4. Return to the front and repeat the twist to the left.

6. The Standing Spinal Twist
(parivrtta trikonasana)

    This posture has been modified for pregnancy but it is the most difficult of the Spinal Twists and for that reason is not suitable for everybody. It is considered to be an invigorating

Asana
Spinal twists

exercise. If you do decide to include it in your yoga program always prepare your body first by loosening your spinal column with one of the other twists first. The benefits for your back are similar to the previous exercises only to a greater degree and your calf muscles and hamstrings are stretched, toned and made more flexible.

Note: This is a head down posture so if you have high or low blood pressure move very slowly through the movements and don't do the twist if it makes you dizzy or uncomfortable.

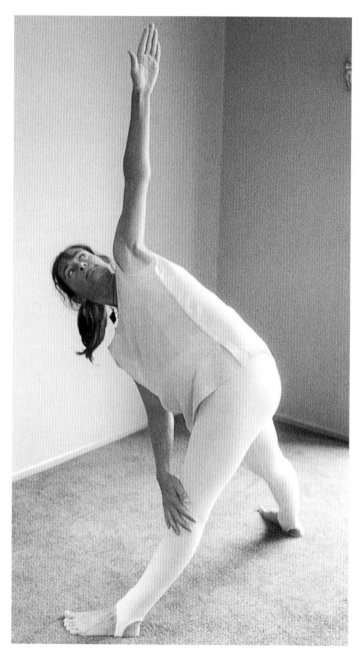

Variation (i)

1. Stand with your feet facing the front, one to one and a half metres apart.

2. Breathe in as you raise your arms out to the sides at shoulder height. Keep your shoulders relaxed.

3. Breathe out and turn your body to the left. Place your right hand on your left leg or left foot. Raise your left arm up high and look at your left hand. Keep your knees straight. Your right hand can rest anywhere on your left leg that is comfortable. Reaching for your foot is only recommended if you are flexible, familiar with the posture and have been practising yoga for some time.

4. Breathe in and return to the standing position.

5. Breathe out as you turn your body to the right. Place your left hand on your right leg or foot, looking up at your right hand. Continue to do this slowly and gently up to five times each side, feeling your body loosen as you proceed with the exercise.

Variation (ii)

If you were quite comfortable with the first variation, you may benefit from holding the final posture while you relax and breathe deeply into the twist. This allows a deeper stretch in your hamstring tendons, leg muscles and lower back. As your head is down for longer, however, return to the standing position slowly to prevent dizziness. Remember to hold the twist for the same length of time on both sides.

When you have completed the posture shake your feet and legs lightly.

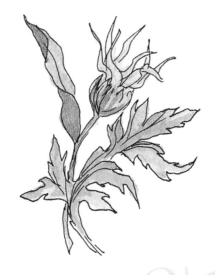

MUDRA
Mudras for Pregnancy

When the word *mudra* is translated from Sanskrit it means an attitude or gesture by a part of your body. It also refers to a part of your body that is sealed or closed off. The prominent Indian yoga teacher, Swami Satyananda (1978), said a *mudra* is: 'a psychic attitude often expressed by a physical gesture, movement or posture which affects the flow of psychic energy in the body.'

In eastern dance *mudras* are found as gestures of the hands, fingers and eyes. The dancer uses these gestures to represent desired moods or feelings. In yoga, many of the *mudras* are quite involved and are only practised by experienced yoga devotees. However, they can also be of the simplest nature, unobtrusive and modest positions of the fingers, eyes and other parts of the body. Even these simple gestures have a profound effect on the mental and spiritual aspects of the person.

I have recommended seven *mudras* for pregnancy. The first four are generally used during meditation, deep relaxation or breathing exercises (*pranayama*). The fifth and sixth are part of advanced yoga practices but still of benefit during pregnancy while the seventh is similar in application and effect to the pelvic floor exercises.

1. & 2. The Psychic Gestures of Consciousness and Knowledge
(chin mudra & gyana mudra)

Chin mudra and *gyana mudra* are very similar to each other and the benefits gained from practising them are also comparable. They are very simple to do and their influence is extremely subtle. It may not be immediately apparent that they are quietening your mind, but with time and patience your awareness will become finely tuned to the delicate energies you possess. You might then find yourself intuitively joining your thumb and first finger as you practise the *asanas* and *pranayama*, meditate or move into deep relaxation.

According to traditional yogic texts, the index finger represents the soul and the thumb represents higher or supreme consciousness. By joining your thumb and first finger an important connection occurs between your soul and your higher consciousness or spiritual energy. The union of your psychic mind and physical nervous system causes impulses from your hands to be directed back into your body as *prana*, or psychic energy.

1. If you are in a seated, cross-legged position for the breathing exercises or for meditation, place your hands on your knees. Join the tips of your thumb and index finger, on each hand. Your other fingers will curl slightly inwards. For *chin mudra*, your palms face up, and for *gyana mudra* your palms face down. For deep relaxation (*yoga nidra*), use *chin mudra*.

3. The Terrifying Attitude
(*bhairava mudra*)

Bhairava mudra is a comfortable and easy way to hold your hands for the breathing exercises, meditation or while resting. It is referred to as the fierce or terrifying attitude of Lord Shiva and the separation or annulment of the universe, but it is, in fact, a very unassuming way of holding your hands. As with the first two *mudras*, your hands represent the individual soul and the supreme consciousness, and likewise a peaceful feeling is encouraged when your hands are in this position.

1. Sit in a comfortable position with your spine straight and your body relaxed. With both palms facing upwards, place your right hand on top of your left. If your left hand is on top of your right hand it is known as *bhairavi mudra*, which is the female equivalent of *bhairava mudra*.

4. The Womb or Source
(*yoni mudra*)

Yoni mudra has particular relevance for women and pregnancy as the word, *yoni*, means womb or source. In Barbara

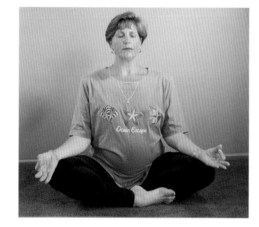

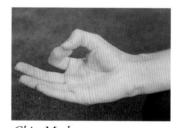

Chin Madra

108

The complete book of
yoga and meditation
for pregnancy

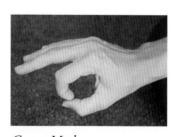

Gyana Mudra

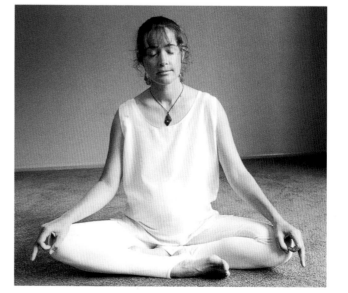

Walker's huge book, *The Woman's Encyclopaedia of Myths and Secrets* (1983), *yoni* is described as being 'the Primordial Image representing the Great Mother as the source of all life.' She goes on to say, 'as the genital focus of her divine energy, the Yoni Yantra was adorned as a geometrical symbol, as the cross was adorned by Christians.'

It is interesting to note that the Sanskrit word for a sanctuary or temple was *garbha-grha*, which means womb when translated. The womb is where life's creation begins and is therefore a sanctuary or temple for human life.

Yoni mudra will bring quietness and stillness to your mind and body. It will also balance the left and right sides of your brain. It is excellent to use when practising breathing exercises and while meditating because it helps to intensify concentration and relaxation.

triangle resembling the shape of the womb, and symbolising the entrance to the womb.

5. The Psychic Union
(yoga mudra)

Yoga mudra is an incredibly peaceful yoga practice and the benefits are noticed almost immediately. It is usually performed as part of an advanced meditation program which focuses on your body's *chakra* system. Although this version has been modified, it still has an extremely calming and centring effect on both the mind and body. It is an excellent preparation for meditation and becoming still, and is therefore an ideal practice for pregnant women. The *ujjayi pranayama* technique is traditionally used in conjunction with these movements so they can also be practised as part of your breathing program.

This posture massages your digestive system, helping to relieve indigestion, constipation and other minor abdominal discomforts. Your back is gently stretched as you move forward, relieving stiffness through your neck, back and shoulders. Your nervous system is balanced and nourished, which helps to calm your emotions. A tendency towards anger and frustration will be relieved and gradually give way to a quieter outlook.

As your head is in a downward position you will tend to relax, and the rocking

1. Sit comfortably with your spine straight, your eyes lightly closed and your body and mind relaxed.

2. With your arms relaxed and your hands resting in your lap, interlock your fingers.

3. Straighten your index fingers and join them together from the top of your finger to the first finger joint. They should be pointing downwards. Join your thumbs together. They should be facing upwards. This will form a

Left:
The Terrifying
Attitude

Below:
The Womb

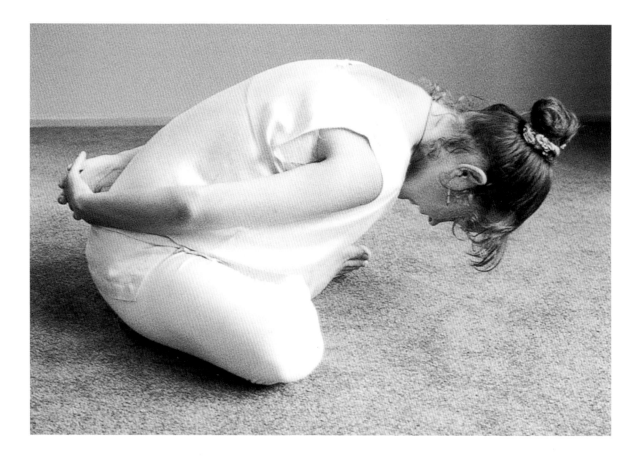

motion brings with it a feeling of peace. These movements, when combined with the *ujjayi* breathing, will very quickly calm you, just as a baby is soothed and quietened by gentle rocking.

1. Sit with your legs in a comfortable cross-legged position, your spine is straight and your eyes lightly closed. The *ujjayi* breathing is preferred for *yoga mudra*, but slow relaxed breathing is also acceptable.

2. Join your hands behind your back with your fingers interlocked and your palms facing up. Relax your arms from your shoulders.

3. Breath in while your body is in an upright position. Breathe out as you move your body forward and lower your head as close to the floor as possible. In the traditional exercise your head would be touching the floor, but during pregnancy you might feel uncomfortable doing this so it is quite acceptable to rock only a little way

forward with each breath. With this modification you will still receive all the benefits without unnecessary discomfort or strain. As you move your body forward make sure that your neck is relaxed and the crown of your head is towards the floor. This will prevent any tightness or tension being held in your shoulders and neck.

4. Continue with this rocking movement and the *ujjayi* breathing up to nine times, or as long as you are enjoying it. You will find that the more you practise the quieter your breathing will become and the more slowly you will rock forward and back, almost as if in a hypnotic trance.

6. Eyebrow Centre Gazing
(shambhavi mudra)

Shambhavi mudra is considered to be one of the most powerful practices for drawing your awareness inwards and is therefore an important preparation

110

The complete book of
yoga and meditation
for pregnancy

for meditation. It has a quietening effect on your mind and induces a more inward perception. It encourages us to recognise a quieter place within ourselves, which is away from the sensory stimuli of our lives. It is part of an advanced yoga study called Kriya Yoga, and is one of the main practices for stimulating and awakening *ajna chakra*, or the eyebrow centre chakra.

Physically, your eyes and the muscles around your eyes are made stronger with regular practice. Mentally, the practice induces calmness and balances your emotions. Concentration is improved, and mental and emotional stability is enhanced. If you wish to explore the spiritual development associated with stimulating the *ajna chakra* it is preferable to seek the assistance of a proficient teacher.

1. Sit on the floor in a comfortable cross-legged position, or in a chair with your spine straight. Your hands can be in any one of the *mudras*. Lightly close your eyes.

2. Open your eyes and focus on a point in front of you. Your head can be tilted back slightly for comfort. Look up towards your eyebrows and then draw your focus in to the point at the centre of your eyebrows. Keep your face and eyes relaxed and if you need to blink, do so. Close your eyes if you feel any strain or discomfort. When you are ready, close your eyes gently.

3. Keep your eyes closed for a short time and then repeat the practice. At first it might be a little uncomfortable to hold the posture for any length of time. With practice it becomes easier and your eyes can be held open for longer. When you close your eyes you will notice a feeling of

lightness, calmness and stillness in your mind.

7. The Horse
(ashwini mudra)

In some texts, the Pelvic Floor exercises are called *ashwini mudra*. However, there are two separate practices which aptly describe the Pelvic Floor exercises; *ashwini mudra* and *moola bandha*. Although there is a slight difference between them, the similarity and benefits become obvious when they are practised in conjunction but as separate exercises. In *ashwini mudra* you tighten your anal area. In *moola bandha* (which I describe in the pelvic floor exercises) you contract your perineum and vaginal areas. Together they become the Pelvic Floor exercises.

When you first try these exercises it might be difficult to isolate one area from the other, but with practice there is a noticeable difference as more control is established.

It can be practised sitting in a chair or in a cross-legged position and, like the pelvic floor exercises, can be done anywhere and at any time without people knowing you are doing them.

The Horse *mudra* is especially useful in helping to prevent constipation and haemorrhoids. As this exercise works so deeply into your pelvic floor area, there is less chance of prolapses and incontinence occurring. Control over your anal sphincter muscles is also improved.

1. Breathe in while lifting and tightening your anus.

2. Hold for a short time before releasing and relaxing as you breathe out. Repeat this as often as required.

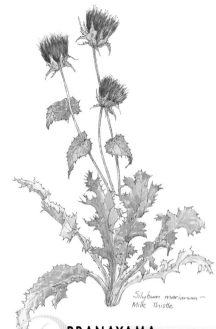
Silybum marianum – Milk Thistle.

PRANAYAMA
Seated postures for Pranayama and Meditation

If you create an auspicious condition in your body and your environment, the meditation and realisation will automatically arise. (Sogyal Rinpoche 1994, p. 32)

Whenever I am practising *pranayama* or meditation, I like to feel still and steady like a mountain. I have incorporated this potent image into my yoga classes and it is amazing how solid, grounded and steady everybody looks. One lady said that whenever she felt unsettled and confused at work, she imagined herself as a mountain, immovable in her centredness and steadiness. I have found that this is a truly valuable concept to have and use in daily life as well as in preparation for birth. In the chapter, 'Meditation', I have included a practice based on this image.

There are five seated postures traditionally used for breathing exercises

(*pranayama*) and meditation, and it is preferable to begin with a posture that is comfortable for you to hold. Spending a little time each day in the easier postures will quickly increase your flexibility and as you feel ready you can include the more challenging postures into your program. The aim is to be able to hold a posture comfortably – during *pranayama* or meditation – without the need to change your position.

In all the postures it is important to hold your spine straight and to keep your body relaxed. Generally, your eyes should be lightly closed, your teeth a little apart and your face relaxed. Keep your arms slightly bent at the elbows to prevent tension in your arms and shoulders.

I recommend that your hands be resting in either *chin mudra, gyana mudra, yoni mudra* or *bhairava mudra*. Before sitting, loosen your feet and hips with a few of the following practices:

112

The complete book of
yoga and meditation
for pregnancy

the Ankle exercises, the Hip Rotation, the Butterfly, Crow Walking and any of the other squatting postures.

Sitting on the floor for any length of time can be a new experience and sometimes quite uncomfortable for many of us, but with a little patience most of the seated postures can be managed and maintained in complete comfort. It is also quite acceptable to sit on a small cushion to help overcome any initial discomfort. Simply place one or two small cushions under your tail bone. This will elevate your lower body and tilt your pelvis slightly forward, allowing your knees to rest closer to the floor. This will enable you to sit with your spine straight and back relaxed for the duration of the practice, while relieving any discomfort or pain in your back.

1. The Easy Posture
(sukhasana)

The Easy Posture is suitable for almost everyone, and is an ideal posture for beginners. Sitting on the floor with your legs crossed may appear easy, but unless you do this regularly you might find it uncomfortable to begin with. With regular practise however this posture often becomes a favourite position.

In this posture, physical steadiness is established, which is necessary for *pranayama* and meditation. Your hips and pelvic areas are loosened and with time they become supple. Your whole back and spinal column are encouraged to remain firm

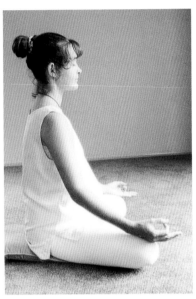

and strong, and with practise your knees and ankles become flexible and loose. Time spent in this posture will establish balance and calmness in your mind and emotions.

1. Begin by sitting on the floor with your legs stretched out in front of

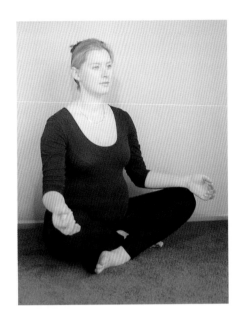

you, and your spine relaxed and straight.

2. Bend your right leg and place your right foot under your left thigh. Place your left foot under your right thigh. Adjust your position until you are completely comfortable, then close your eyes. This posture can be held for as long as desired. When you have completed the practice, unfold your legs and shake them lightly.

2. The Adept's Posture
(siddhasana)

In this posture your knees will come closer to the floor than in the Easy Posture, and with practice this can be managed by most people. The benefits are similar to the previous posture only more flexibility is encouraged in your hips and pelvis.

1. Begin in the Easy Posture, then pull your right heel in against your

Pranayama
Seated postures for pranayama
and meditation

perineum or as close to your pelvic floor as possible.

2. Place your left heel in front of your right ankle. In this posture your knees will be close to the floor as your pelvic muscles extend and relax. Relax your whole body, and keep your eyes lightly closed.

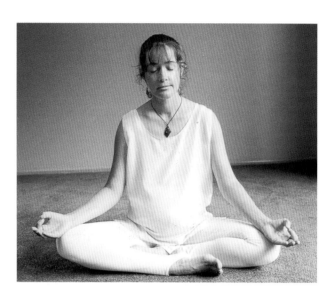

3. The Half Lotus
(ardha padmasana)

Padma means lotus, and this posture is a good preparation for the Lotus posture. It is best practised when the easier seated postures have been mastered.

1. Sit with your legs in front of you. Place your right foot on top of your left thigh. Rest your left foot beside your right inner thigh, as close to your groin as possible. This can be reversed to gain flexibility in both ankles and legs. Lightly close your eyes. Hold the posture for as long as you are comfortable. When you release your legs from the posture, shake them lightly.

4. The Lotus
(padmasana)

This posture is one of the most well recognised and important in yoga. For many, it is the posture of choice for

meditation and advanced *pranayama*, and once mastered it brings balance and stability to both mind and body. It is not the easiest of postures to become accustomed to but with regular practice will eventually be achieved. I recommend you practise the Half Lotus and feel comfortable in that posture before attempting the Lotus.

The Lotus will bring stillness and steadiness to your whole body by balancing and relaxing your nervous

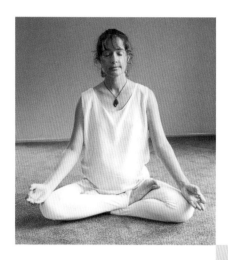

system. Practitioners of this posture realise mental clarity, emotional calmness and physical stillness. Stiffness is removed from your knees, hips and ankles and circulation is improved to your lower back and pelvis. As there is a greater blood supply to your abdominal area, this posture is also beneficial for your digestive system and reproductive system. Your spine is encouraged to remain erect and steady, which creates the correct atmosphere for the flow of vital energy *(prana)* up and down your spine.

Before commencing the Lotus, loosen and relax your feet and your ankles by practising the Ankle exercises.

1. Sit on the floor with your legs in front of you and your spine straight.

2. Bend your right leg and place your right foot on top of your left

114

The complete book of
yoga and meditation
for pregnancy

thigh, as close to your groin as possible.

3. Bend your left leg and place your left foot in your right thigh. Move your knees as close to the floor as possible. Your heels need to be as close as possible to your pelvis, and the soles of your feet facing upwards. Your eyes should be lightly closed. Hold the posture for as long as you are comfortable. When you release your legs from the posture, shake them lightly.

At no time force your legs into the Lotus posture. It needs to be remembered that many yoga postures are unfamiliar to your body and it takes patience and time for the muscles to become free and loose enough to achieve the postures comfortably. So it is important to always approach the postures in a gentle manner.

5. The Breath Balancing Posture
(padadhirasana)

When you practise *pranayama*, you might notice that one nostril is more blocked than the other. By placing your fingertips under your armpits, the flow of air through both nostrils will be normalised. At the same time, the right and left sides of your brain become balanced, creating a calmer state of mind. This is because there are pressure points under your armpits, which relate to the opposite nostrils. For example, your right nostril is cleared by placing your right hand or fingertips under your left armpit, and vice versa.

Take note of which nostril is clear when you are relaxed and your mind is free. Most probably it will be your left nostril which corresponds to the quieter and less analytical right side of your brain. This is worthwhile remembering when you are having trouble sleeping because by lying on your right side the flow of air will increase in your left nostril and stimulate the right side of

your brain. The reverse is also true if you need to 'wake up' or think more clearly. Then it is your right nostril which needs to be flowing freely.

Any time you need to be still and centred, this posture will very quickly and gently help to establish a quieter atmosphere in your mind, and I feel it would be an ideal practice to do in the early moments of labour.

You might have noticed people standing in conversation with their arms crossed over their chest in this manner. Some would say it is body language suggesting protection or covering of the heart centre. This may be true, but I feel it is because we instinctively know that when we have our arms crossed in this way we are relaxed and balanced and therefore more likely to have a calm and pleasant conversation.

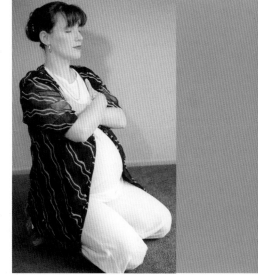

1. Sit in the Thunderbolt posture or one of the other seated postures. Your spine needs to be straight, and your eyes lightly closed.

2. Cross your arms in front of your chest making sure that your right arm is in front of your left. Place your fingertips into your armpits. Keep your thumbs on the outside of your armpits, facing up. Relax your shoulders.

3. Concentrate on breathing quietly, and stay in this posture for 10 minutes or longer. You will notice that the longer you remain in this posture the slower your breathing will become and the more relaxed you will feel. I often suggest practising the *ujjayi pranayama* while sitting in this posture because one practice really complements the other.

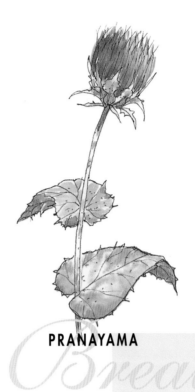

PRANAYAMA

Breathing

Life is the interval between one breath and another – he who only breathes half, only lives half. But he who master[s] the art of breathing has control over every function of his being.
(Shri Yogendra 1977, p. 17)

The word *prana* means energy, vitality, wind, life force and respiration. It is said that; 'No greater element than bioenergy (Prana) exists in the body.' (Yogendra 1977, p. 17). The word yama means to control. Therefore, the practice of *pranayama* is to control the vital energy and life force that is within each breath. It also means, utilising this energy to its fullest capacity as it flows through the body.

Breathing is a completely natural process that is mostly unconscious from the moment that we take our first breath at birth until the last breath leaves the body at our death. However, through the practice of *pranayama*, we gradually become more conscious of the movements of our breathing, witnessing and observing its rhythmic, steady and balanced flow. The practice of *pranayama* is so vital to our wellbeing that to practise yoga without it is to realise only a fraction of yoga's extraordinary potential and possibilities.

When we breathe more efficiently it ensures a healthy blood flow to the brain so that the mind remains clear and is free from mental confusion. During moments of stress, our breathing usually becomes rapid, shallow and high in the chest. This rapid, shallow breathing results in less oxygen circulating around your body and reaching your brain. A stress cycle is then created resulting in diminished clarity and sometimes confused or irrational behaviour.

If, however, we can somehow remove ourselves from the moment, witness the way we are breathing and remember to breathe slowly and deeply we could also create the space for more logical thinking. We can then distance ourselves from the situation, be more clearly in the present moment and manage our response in a more acceptable way. Of course, this is easier said than done but many people notice a difference in the way they manage stressful situations as they develop control of their breathing.

One of the main purposes of *pranayama* is to feel quiet and still. Over time, you will become more skilled at the practices, and others will notice a difference in your energy as you become a little more relaxed and your life somehow seems slower and less hectic. You will become quietly more aware and observant of aspects of your life. Just as we now realise how important it is to exercise, it is also of extreme value to discipline ourselves to breathe more efficiently. The more time spent becoming familiar with the breathing exercises, the better you will feel, physically, mentally and emotionally.

Preparation

Before practising *pranayama* it is important to be aware of the following points:

1. Always practise under the guidance of a teacher who is well experienced and knowledgeable in yoga breathing exercises. In this way if any problems arise they can be quickly corrected.

2. If you feel light headed or faint, it is important to discontinue with the practice until you restore balance in your body. Although this is not a common problem, it does occur occasionally due to an increased oxygen uptake by your body's circulatory system.

3. Always proceed slowly and gradually for the best results.

4. It is important to be in a comfortable seated position. Your spine should be straight and your body relaxed. The preferred postures are described in the chapter, 'Seated Postures for Pranayama & Meditation'. If you find them hard to manage you may sit with your back against a wall and your legs straight out in front, or sit in a straight-backed chair with your legs uncrossed and your feet flat on the floor.

5. When you do your yoga *asanas* or other exercises, try to leave some time for the breathing practices, too. As I have suggested in the 'Introduction', the breathing exercises can be practised after the *asana*s and before meditation and relaxation. In this way you will be completing a balanced program.

6. To begin with, allow about five to ten minutes for *pranayama*. Over time this can be increased to meet your own specific needs. Keep each breath flowing evenly and smoothly in and out of your body – never 'jerking' your breathing – and at no time becoming breathless. Remember not to strain your breath in an effort to complete an exercise. Keep in mind that the practices are gentle and designed to have a calming and relaxing effect.

7. During pregnancy it is not advisable to hold your breath for a long time but rather to keep your breath flowing evenly in and out of your body. A short breath retention is acceptable when you are proficient with the breathing practices, however, this needs to be taught under the guidance of an experienced teacher.

8. Your body needs to be completely relaxed and free of all tension. Have your eyes lightly closed, your teeth a little apart and your jaw relaxed. Your hands can be placed on your knees with the palms facing down or in one of the *mudra*s (see Contents).

It is best to have your arms slightly bent to prevent tension building up in your arms and shoulders.

9. Before commencing the breathing exercises, spend a few quiet moments following your natural breath and clearing your mind so that you feel calm, still and centred before beginning.

10. Practise in a well-ventilated room, away from outside disturbances and excess noise. If you can, take the phone off the hook and let others know you would appreciate some time on your own to practise your yoga breathing.

11. Wear loose comfortable clothing. Your body temperature will drop as you become more relaxed, so it is useful to cover your shoulders with a light rug before you begin and wear socks if your feet are inclined to get cold easily.

12. If possible, practise before eating. If this is not possible eat a light snack instead of a full meal. Whenever possible, your bladder and bowels should be emptied before starting.

13. Before you begin your breathing exercises, practise the Heavenly Stretch posture (see the chapter 'Standing') and some of the other exercises where your arms are lifted above your head and your chest is expanded. This encourages more efficient breathing and also prepares your lungs for the breathing exercises. Refer to the sections 'Standing' and 'Warming up', for details of these exercises.

14. Deep breathing is not recommended for people with high blood pressure or heart problems. If you have one of these problems, proceed by slow degrees and under experienced supervision so that your body becomes accustomed to these practices gently and safely.

Caution: If you feel light-headed or notice a shortness of breath, stop the practice until your breathing has equalised.

1. The Complete Breath

The value of the Complete Breath – or Deep Yoga Breathing as it is also called – cannot be overemphasised as the whole person benefits in a dynamic and positive way. The middle of your body – or your solar plexus – is often referred to as the emotional centre of our physical body. It tightens and 'closes up' when we are feeling unsettled emotionally, for example in times of fear, anxiety or anger. Before people learn to breathe from a yogic point of view, they are generally not using the full capacity of their lungs and therefore have a much diminished uptake and utilisation of oxygen throughout the body.

Most people breathe in a very shallow manner where the breath is light and short within the chest cavity and the muscles of the chest and upper/middle back are never fully expanded. This means that they never reach full breath volume and lung capacity while either breathing in or out.

We can divide the cycle of a breath into three parts; the inhalation, the retention of the breath (which for pregnancy is kept to a minimum), and the exhalation. For the purposes of the pregnant woman, the incoming and outgoing breaths should be equal in length. You will notice that with regular practice your breath becomes longer, deeper and slower as your lungs are encouraged to expand more completely, while the whole respiratory system is strengthened and assisted to work more efficiently.

The complete book of
yoga and meditation
for pregnancy

The incoming breath can be used to replenish you with all the healing qualities that you need to maintain balance and harmony on all levels. The outgoing breath can be used to release any tension and stress from your body and your mind. In this way you are using the breath and the power of your thoughts to create the feelings most needed at the time. This concept can be applied to drawing in energy and vitality if you are fatigued, and to releasing weariness as you breathe out. Likewise, you can draw in peace and stillness and calmness when you feel anxious or stressed. Colour can be used in the same way for the purposes of healing by either drawing it into a particular part of the body, to the whole body or to surround the body.

Abdominal breathing is where your abdomen is gently pushed out, allowing the base of your lungs to expand and fill with air. To begin with, exaggerate this movement so as to really feel your abdominal area working. Keep the emphasis on moving these muscles out from your body rather than drawing them inwards. By placing your fingertips together on your navel you will notice your fingers move apart when you inhale and as you exhale they come together again. When abdominal breathing is done correctly, your navel appears to lift as you breathe in and fall back into your body as you breathe out.

This type of breathing has many advantages and can be used where there is tightness or cramping in your pelvic region, helping to relax and open the muscles of this area.

Thoracic breathing is where your breath is taken deeply into your upper chest for a full expansion of your chest. Your shoulders will lift slightly and your whole upper body is expanded as your lungs push your rib cage wide. When exhaling, the muscles of your chest relax, your abdominal area moves back into your body and your chest contracts. This is often described as being similar to the movement of a slow wave moving out to sea and then back

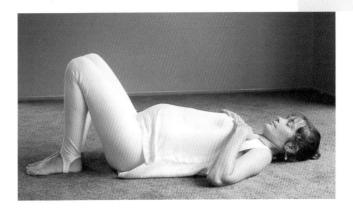

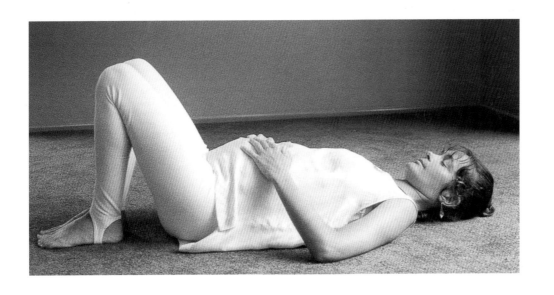

into the shore, an image which is described more fully in the Ocean of Abundance visualisation in the chapter, 'Visualisations & Creative Meditations'. Your body lifts and expands while breathing in, and contracts and relaxes as you breathe out. If your fingertips are placed together in the middle of your chest, you will notice them move slightly apart as you breathe in, coming together again as you breathe out. This whole movement is slow and controlled without any strain or shortness of breath.

Deep yoga breathing is where abdominal breathing and thoracic breathing are combined to make a slow full breath, and it involves a complete expansion and contraction of your lungs.

At the initiation of the breath your abdomen is expanded outwards, allowing your diaphragm to move down and the base of your lungs to expand. Your breath then continues slowly to fill your middle and upper chest. It's as if there is a deflated balloon inside your body, which begins to inflate with air as your breath is drawn into your abdomen, and then deflates as your lungs empty with a full exhalation.

When you breathe out, gently push the last remaining air from your lungs so that you feel your abdomen flatten slightly. I emphasise this point because a lot of people breathe in deeply but don't seem to breathe out so completely. Remember to always breathe in and out evenly to maintain equilibrium throughout your whole body.

I suggest that people begin by completing only three deep yoga breaths at a time, and repeating that procedure three times a day. When you become familiar with the exercise, this number can be increased to five breaths or more.

With regular practice you will notice your breath becoming longer and deeper as your lungs expand more completely.

2. Alternate Nostril Breath
(nadi shodhana)

Alternate Nostril Breathing is one of the most important *pranayama* practices and is also one of the most frequently used. It is highly recommended for the health of the mind and the emotions, and is an excellent preparation for meditation because it quietens the mind and very

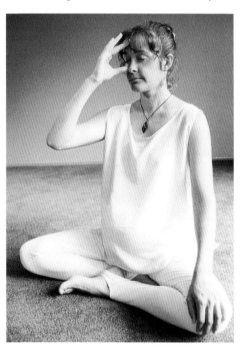

quickly establishes stillness in the body.

The benefits of the Alternate Nostril Breath are threefold. Firstly, from a physical perspective, this practice will help balance the left and right sides of your brain as the breath flows evenly through both nostrils.

It is an excellent practice for the respiratory system, assisting in toning and strengthening the lungs and airways. Oxygen is more efficiently taken in with the breath and carbon dioxide is removed as the breath is encouraged to be even and harmonious.

As the lungs are one of the major pathways of elimination in the body, toxins are also more efficiently removed from the body.

This form of breathing also greatly benefits those who tend to breathe 'shallow' or through their mouth, and sinus congestion is removed as the breath is encouraged to flow equally in and out of the nostrils.

Secondly, your mind is prevented from wandering as your awareness and concentration are focused on controlling the even flow of breath through the individual nostrils. Your awareness comes more into the present moment, establishing both mental and emotional stability and the physical action of this breathing exercise induces tranquillity and an overall sense of calmness.

The third benefit of this breathing technique is that it creates the right 'atmosphere' for meditation because a total purifying and cleansing of the body and mind takes place with the practice of *nadi shodhana pranayama*.

The word *nadi* refers to a passage where *prana* is able to flow freely. As I have discussed more fully in the chapter, 'What is yoga?', the *nadis* are channels for carrying energy from the spiritual body to the physical body. *Shodhana* means to purify or cleanse. Therefore, by practising *nadi shodhana*, our energy currents – both physical and spiritual – are cleansed and purified.

In yoga philosophy, the left nostril is related to the *ida nadi* and the right nostril to the *pingala nadi*. The breath in the left nostril is cool and corresponds to the moon, also known as *chandra nadi*. The breath in the right nostril is considered hot like the sun, and is known as *surya nadi*. Down the centre of the body is the *sushumna nadi* which is considered to be the most

important *nadi*. The breathing exercises are one of the many ways of balancing and 'recharging' the *nadis* and the *pranic* body.

If one or both of your nostrils is blocked, use the Breath Balancing Posture from the chapter, 'Seated Postures for Pranayama & Meditation', to free up the flow of air.

Variation (i)

1. Sit in a comfortable position with your spine straight and your body relaxed. Using your right hand, place your thumb beside your right nostril, your first two fingers between your eyebrows, and your ring finger beside your left nostril.

2. Block your right nostril with your thumb, and breathe slowly and evenly in and out of your left nostril, three times.

3. Change fingers, blocking your left nostril with your ring finger, and breathe three times in and out of your right nostril. If you are quite comfortable with this number, you can continue on to do nine breaths through the individual nostrils. Always do the same number of breaths through each nostril.

This breathing is meant to be slow, even and controlled. There should not be any discomfort or difficulty. Practice this variation for at least two weeks or until you become confident and relaxed with it, then advance to Variation (ii).

Variation (ii)

1. Begin with your hand in the same position as for Variation (i).

2. With your right nostril blocked, breathe in though your left nostril.

3. Change fingers by releasing your right nostril, block your left nostril

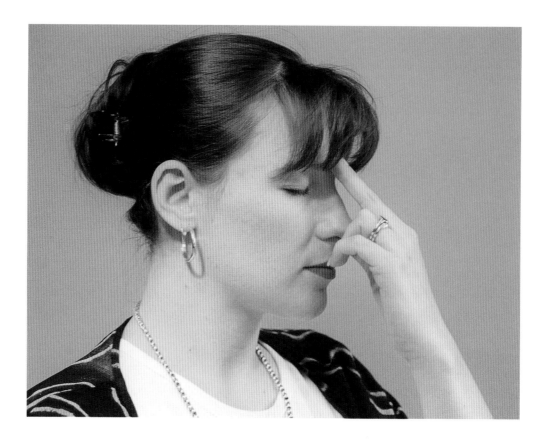

Alternate Nostril Breath

and breathe out through your right nostril.

4. Breathe in through your right nostril, change fingers and breathe out through your left nostril. Explained more simply, breathe in through your left nostril, out through your right, in through your right and out through your left. This completes one round of the Alternate Nostril Breath.

5. Repeat this four more times to complete five rounds altogether. Try to breathe in and out evenly at all times. Do not hold your breath or alter the breathing pattern in any way.

3. The Cooling Breath
(sheetali pranayama)

Over the years of recommending different breathing exercises for labour, I have found there are many women who have successfully used the Cooling Breath to help them remain centred and calm after a contraction. It also helped them restore lost energy from one

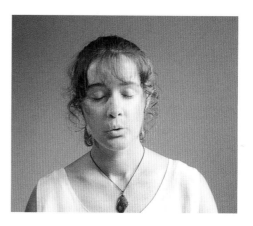

contraction to the next. Other women spoke of how it helped to take their minds away from being fearful or anxious, and to stay focused on the present moment, enabling them to remain in a space of peace. It is a simple exercise involving very little effort other than feeling the coolness of your breath over your tongue as you breathe in.

It becomes an even more powerful technique when specific visualisations or images are used in conjunction with the breath. For example, before you begin to practise,

122

The complete book of
yoga and meditation
for pregnancy

bring to mind what your needs are at that moment. Maybe you are feeling drained and fatigued because of a long and difficult labour and it is energy you are needing. At another time you might feel a need to fill yourself with light, peace and calmness. You may also visualise a specific colour that expresses your needs at that time. Draw these qualities into your body as you breathe in.

Another very useful technique is to imagine your own special place in nature. Somewhere that makes you feel quiet and calm. This might be somewhere in the world you have never been to, but just the idea of this place has the same calming effect on you. Imagine these powerful yet gentle energies being drawn into your body, your mind and your spirit with each breath. These principles are suitable for all the breathing exercises but especially with *sheetali*, where you can feel the cool stream of air passing over your tongue as you breathe in.

Sheetali pranayama cools your body and has a stabilising effect on your blood pressure, making it a valuable choice if your blood pressure is high or low. It is also said to be one of the most efficient ways of directing *prana* throughout your body or to specific parts of your body. With regular practice the blood becomes purified and your body will feel still and relaxed.

There are two variations of the Cooling Breath, one with your tongue relaxed in your mouth and the other with your tongue curled. Some people are genetically unable to curl their tongue and will find the second variation impossible.

1. With your mouth in the shape of an 'O', as if you are going to whistle, breathe in slowly while feeling the cool stream of air over your tongue.

2. Close your mouth and breathe out through your nose. Repeat this up to nine times. Your breath can either be at your regular breathing pace or a slower, deeper breath. Sometimes repeating too many Cooling Breaths will make you thirsty, so if you plan to use this technique during labour, sip a little water every so often.

3. If you can curl your tongue, open your mouth, curl your tongue and breathe in feeling the air channelled through the tunnel shape of your tongue. Close your mouth and breathe out through your nose.

4. The Hissing Breath
(sheetkari pranayama)

The Hissing Breath is similar in procedure and benefits to the Cooling Breath. The only difference is the position of your mouth and tongue. Some people prefer this exercise, as they feel it provides a greater volume of cool air.

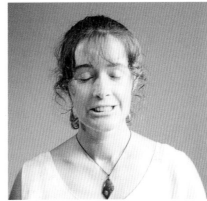

1. With your teeth together and your lips slightly open, breathe in slowly and deeply.

2. Close your mouth and breathe out through your nose. Repeat this nine times.

5. The Humming Breath
(bhramari pranayama)

The word *bhramari* means large black bee and when this exercise is done correctly the sound you make is similar to that of a bee. For some people it takes a little while to perfect this practice and produce a continuous, even sound and hum with the exhalation.

The word 'om' is well known in yoga philosophy and also to many other spiritual sources. Dr Wayne Dyer (1997) speaks at length about sound and healing in his book *Manifest Your Destiny*. He says that sounds 'are a powerful healing energy. Every sound is a vibration made of waves oscillating at a particular frequency. . . Sound has healing properties when it is harmonious and soothing.' (Dyer 1997, p. 113).

The word om is often said to represent the sound of the universe or the sound of God. The Humming Breath is like the 'm' sound of om. When I do this breathing exercise, I like to imagine the healthy cells in my body being enlivened, and any 'off colour' cells being either restored or eliminated. It is interesting to note that Dyer also mentions that women of ancient times apparently used the sound of om while birthing their babies (Dyer 1997, p. 114). Maybe now with the use of the Humming Breath, women will once more reconnect with their innate knowing and wisdom.

In the middle of reviewing the Humming Breath, I received a phone call from a woman in my class, called Lynn. Lynn had just given birth to a boy called, Koen. She had been coming to yoga since the 12th week of her pregnancy, and when she was first introduced to the Humming Breath she liked it immediately.

She told me that during the labour she used this exercise along with her birth support people, and found she was able to breathe down into her body, humming louder the more intense the contractions became.

Listening to her own sound through each contraction enabled her to create the concentration and balance she needed.

As already mentioned, this exercise will help to initiate balance throughout your whole body and mind because of the soothing vibrations the sound creates. It is an excellent way to clear the mind of unwanted thoughts because it is difficult to concentrate on thinking while you are humming. Even if you *are* still able to think while you hum – as some people are – when this technique is practised for the recommended time, your mind becomes gradually quieter and more centred. This benefits the nervous system and puts you in touch with your 'inner being'. It is highly recommended for those times when you feel frustrated, anxious or angry, and it is particularly good for insomnia and extreme restlessness. It's worth remembering that people don't usually hum when they are angry or depressed.

When you hum continuously for three or four minutes, the silence that is experienced afterwards is one of pure peace and tranquillity. You might like to try this on a beach or in a quiet forest, humming for a while and then listening to the sounds all around you. Sometimes, in my yoga classes we do a sound meditation where I ask the class to hum om 27 times or more. When they stop the stillness is almost deafening and the atmosphere in the room is very serene. The value this meditation has for the whole person is exceptional and unlimited.

Everyone will have their own unique humming sound that will resonate with perfect harmony for that person. Some people will hum deep and long, while others will hum a lot higher. When you are breathing slowly and deeply with your full awareness on maintaining a long gentle humming sound it's almost as if you become one with that sound or with *nada* the

124

The complete book of
yoga and meditation
for pregnancy

psychic sound. Become aware of feeling its resonance, creating pure stillness and health within every cell of your body, in every thought and in all your emotions. Your thoughts, feelings and physical body become the continuous movement of sound that seems to echo within you and all around you. If you do this regularly during pregnancy, your baby will recognise your special sound after the birth. For the singers among you, the Humming Breath is also recommended for improving your voice and strengthening your throat.

1. Sit in a comfortable position with your spine straight, either cross-legged or in another comfortable position where you can concentrate.

2. Close your eyes and block your ears with your fingers.

3. Breathe in and then out through your nose, making a humming sound as you exhale. Concentrate on the humming sound which will seem to become very loud inside your head when your ears are blocked.

4. Continue for nine breaths or longer. Keep your breathing regular.

This same exercise can also be practised without blocking your ears. In this case, rest your hands on your knees or in one of the mudras.

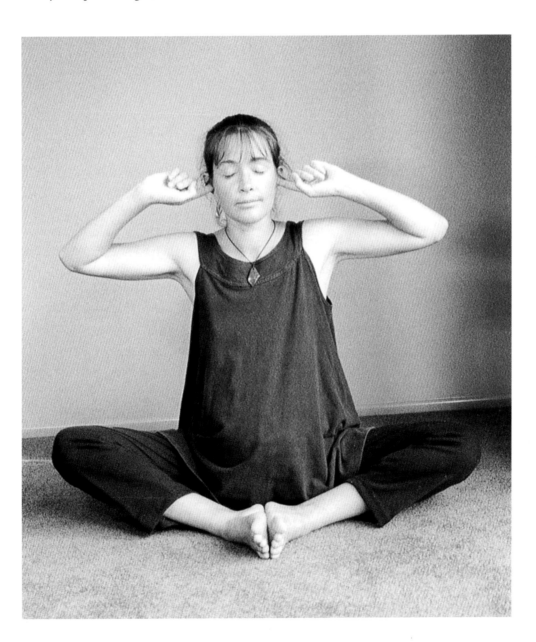

6. The Breath of Tranquillity
(ujjayi pranayama)

The Breath of Tranquillity is sometimes called the Psychic Breath and is one of the most valuable exercises in yoga, and can be used in many situations and circumstances throughout the day. It is known as the Breath of Tranquillity because of the quietening effect it has on the mind, and the Psychic Breath because it leads the practitioner into the more subtle, spiritual aspects of the self. It draws the awareness into a silent place deep within our souls where complete stillness is ever present. We experience a feeling of complete oneness and peace with the inner self, as if time does not exist and where there are no boundaries to prevent us from being at peace.

When the *ujjayi* breathing is practised it's as if we have stepped into eternity. When it is practised for longer periods, such as during meditation, we move beyond limitations to the vast eternal space of the mind, known in yoga as the *chitta kash*.

I feel that it is like looking into the sky which has no beginning or end, just endless space. Close your eyes for a moment, and imagine extending your consciousness out through that space, away from all the activities of your life. You will begin to sense a feeling of incredible silence and stillness. The further you go, the more profound the sensation becomes.

Many of us search for external paths through which to bring quietness and order into our lives. But, if we turn our attention inwards – if we contemplate, meditate and be silent – we find that the peace we seek is within us. Meditation can be explained as 'the art of being still', and the *ujjayi* breathing will initiate that feeling either when practiced as a breathing exercise

or if used for the purpose of meditation. It can be done with the resting breath or in time it can be incorporated into deeper yoga breathing for a more profound result. It is quite a wonderful experience to spend an unlimited time practising the *ujjayi* breathing, observing it becoming slower and quieter the deeper you move into meditation.

Although this is a very gentle breathing exercise, some people are inclined to try too hard. If you strain and force your breath you will find the exercise difficult to do. The sound created has been described as similar to breathing through a hole at the back of your throat. Others explain it as a soft snore, or as like a sleeping baby's breathing. You will notice this sound as you breathe in and out, as well as feeling a slight 'drawing' or tight sensation at the back of your throat.

This exercise helps lower blood pressure. It is acceptable to practise this exercise while lying down, making it an ideal practice if you wake at night and are unable to go back to sleep. Spending some time following the ujjayi breath in the quietness of the night, will often put you back to sleep very quickly. It is also a perfect practice for those new to meditation, as your concentration can be focused on the sound of your breath and the sensation of air in your throat. An *ujjayi* breath is usually longer and deeper than a natural breath, and the more time spent practising this technique the slower you will breathe.

1. Begin by sitting with your spine straight, your body relaxed and your eyes lightly closed. Place your hands in one of the *mudras* or rest them on your knees. Concentrate for a moment on feeling the light sensation of the breath in your nostrils.

2. Continue to breathe in and

126

The complete book of
yoga and meditation
for pregnancy

out through your nose, but now direct your breath towards the back of your throat. If this is difficult to do, concentrate on where your breath is felt in your nostrils. When you are ready, again move your concentration away from your nostrils, as if bypassing them, until you feel as if you are breathing at your throat. When you do this correctly, you will feel a slight tightening sensation at the back of your throat and you will be able to hear the 'drawing' sound.

3. Continue on in this manner for as long as desired. Keep your whole attention on your breathing. You will notice your breath becoming longer and deeper without having to make a conscious effort.

7. The Cleansing Breath
This exercise is not a traditional yoga exercise, but there is a similar exercise done from a standing position where the same principle is applied. This exercise is done in the same way as the Deep Yoga Breathing, the only difference is that the exhalation is through your mouth instead of your nose.

The Cleansing Breath has a powerful influence when your attention is not only on your breathing but also on the concept of blowing away any discomfort in your body, unwanted thoughts or confusion. Bring your attention to those tight or tense parts of your body or unwanted thoughts or uncomfortable feelings and imagine you're blowing them away as you breathe out strongly through your mouth. In this way your breath and your conscious awareness are acting to cleanse your body and mind.

A woman once told me this technique helped her when a bothersome person was invading her space. She was able to 'clear' her space by 'blowing' the person away to a comfortable distance, making the situation easier for her to handle. Although this might sound a bit unusual, it's an extremely effective technique, and many others have used it.

1. Breathe in deeply and slowly through your nose, then breathe out strongly and completely through your mouth as if you are blowing something away. This clears carbon dioxide from your lungs and encourages your body to relax.

2. Keep your attention not only on your breathing but also on the concept of blowing discomfort, unwanted thoughts, confusion or negative emotions away from your body. Use your breath and your conscious awareness together to cleanse your body and mind.

3. Repeat this three or four times, or as many times as you are comfortable with.

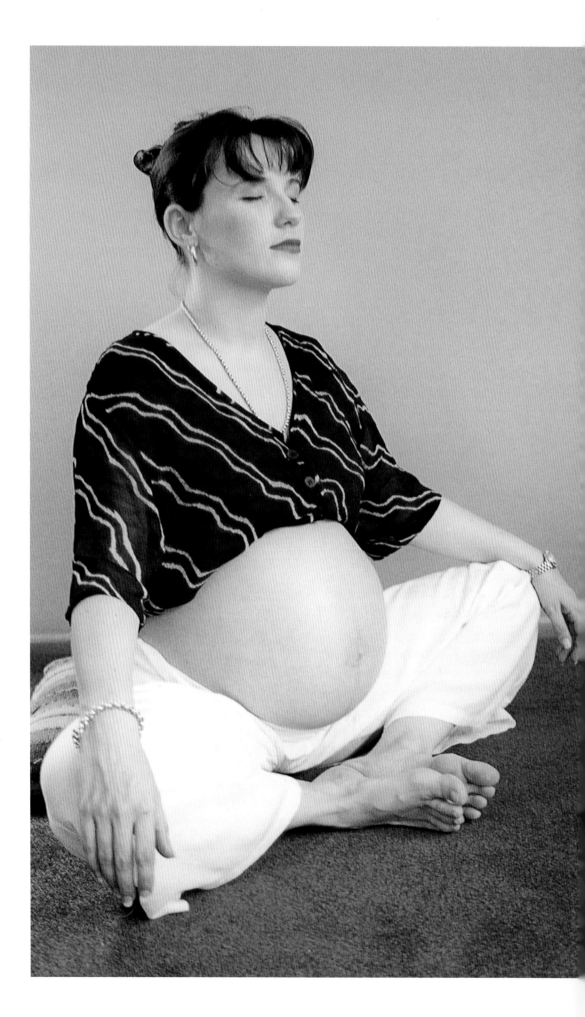

The complete book of
yoga and meditation
for pregnancy

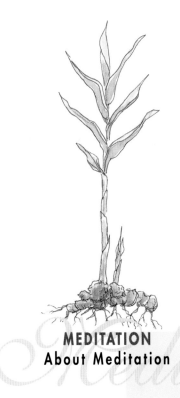

MEDITATION
About Meditation

The controlled mind is conducive to happiness.
Gautama Buddha
(in Sogyal Rinpoche 1994a)

When the time came to write this chapter I found it to be a momentous and all encompassing task. Endeavouring to explain the feeling that is actually experienced during meditation was challenging and awesome. This is because meditation is complex and in many ways beyond words yet at the same time it is a state of pure simplicity in the truest sense. It is the art of being still. Even though I practise meditation as part of my daily life and teach it a number of times each week when it came to putting it in an easy to understand format I found this very simplicity a stumbling block!

What is meditation?

Concentration. Contemplation. Mindfulness. Inner stillness. One pointed awareness. Reflection. Pure awareness. How does one really explain what meditation is or accurately capture its absolute nature? It is as simple as watching the wind moving gently in the trees and yet as complex as understanding why we are here. There are whole books dedicated to this fascinating topic explaining the origins, the different teaching and techniques, how to do it and where to do it, as well as the unlimited benefits it has for the mind and the body. I don't intend to go into such thorough detail here but instead I will keep it as clear and simple as I can. Essentially, that is what meditation really is – clear and simple.

There are many different forms of meditation and many ways to approach it. What you choose to do is obviously a very personal journey, just as inner reflection and time spent alone with yourself is a private concern. However, no matter what path you feel is best for you the various techniques and methods available will eventually lead you to the same place where you come to view and realise the world within – to be alone and at peace with yourself. It is like coming home to yourself. As Sogyal Rinpoche (1994a) says 'Meditation, then, is bringing the mind home.'

Some people come to meditation assuming the mind should be completely free of thought. The mind, however, is rarely completely clear. Thoughts are continually drifting in and out of your mind in the same way that fish swim back and forth in a pond. Sometimes a crab disturbs the mud at the bottom of the pool and the water becomes cloudy, just as disturbance can cause confusion and unsettled thoughts which disturb the clarity in the mind. (Wimala 1998) In time however the mud settles, the water clears and the fish become visible again. It is important to expect nothing from the practice but rather focus on the process of meditating.

When there is an understanding of meditation – where you are the observer and the witness to your total self – all the other yoga practices and techniques are enhanced tenfold. For example, whenever you are practising a yoga posture and you do it with a clear mind that is supremely held in the present moment, you are then more fully aware of being completely in touch with how your body is feeling and the rhythm of your breathing. This prevents mental distraction, physical overextension and straining, so that your yoga postures become a graceful meditation in motion. In this way, meditation can be practised when seated in a cross-legged position or incorporated into every waking moment.

Meditation can be there when you are doing your postures;

mindfulness and inner reflection can be there when you are practising *pranayama*; and present moment awareness can be there when you are relaxing, working, driving the car or watching a film. Every moment is an opportunity to consciously be here, now; in other words, to meditate.

Knowing how to meditate and observe yourself so you are truly living in the now, makes each moment one to remember and enables you to live your life with joy in every moment. This is a point worth considering as no one knows when their last moment will be. Being conscious of this moment, now, as if it was our last, is enough to make sure it is one you are fully aware of and hopefully one that is as joyful as possible.

The gift of learning to meditate is the greatest gift you can give yourself in this life. For it is only through meditation that you can undertake the journey to discover your true nature, and so find the stability and confidence you will need to live and die, well.

(Sogyal Rinpoche 1994a)

All aspects of yoga are important for the pregnant woman. However, without knowing how to be still and at peace with yourself, the other yoga practices seem to have far less impact and value. Whenever I speak to a woman after a birth I ask which aspects of yoga helped the most. It is predominantly the ability to concentrate and focus attention on breathing and on what is happening which proves the most helpful. Familiarity with meditation, mindfulness and present moment awareness enables women to stay focused and centred even during the more intense moments of labour. Through knowledge of simple concentration skills, women are able to be conscious of the birthing process, without feeling dazed, confused or distracted by chaotic moments.

When you are not distracted by a difficult situation your calmness affects others around you. A number of women have told me how valuable they found this practice as they prepared for a caesarean delivery, as it helped them to remain calm before and during the procedure. Because these women were not stressed or anxious about the forthcoming procedure their birth support people were more relaxed too and therefore in a better position to assist and comfort them. It's like a pebble being thrown in the middle of a pond, whose ripples spread unendingly to the edges of the water. If you, as the centre, can be in a state of peaceful calm it will positively affect all those who are there with you.

The meditation practices I have outlined are divided into two groups. The first are traditional meditations from some of the great teachers of past and present times and concentrate on the mind, the senses, the breath and the body. The second group is made up of creative meditations and visualisation techniques which can be used in conjunction with the first group or as separate practices on their own. Some of the practices will appeal to you more than others and will give you excellent results every time. You might be quite content to stay with what is working or you might prefer to experiment by doing a different practice each time.

All the practices are uncomplicated and easy to learn from a book. Obviously, there are some outstanding traditional yoga meditation techniques to be explored but I feel they are best taught on a one-to-one basis from teacher to student. I have found that when meditation is kept straightforward and reasonably simple –

where the technique is in many ways a part of your own nature – the results are always encouraging and more quickly recognised. When you become familiar with the suggestions here you might like to create your own meditations by combining your favourite exercises.

When the time comes for your baby to be born, you will be able to use a number of the exercises to help you stay calm and relaxed, with your awareness in the present moment. The more accustomed and skilled you become with these practices during pregnancy, the more easily they will come to mind during labour. They will become second nature to you and you will instinctively know what will help you the most. I have known many women who practised yoga and meditation consistently during their pregnancies who found themselves automatically doing their most favoured techniques during labour, to their great benefit and relief.

Concentration is the practice whereby one's ordinary, distracted, uncontrolled mind is developed to the point that it can remain powerfully, effortlessly, and one-pointedly on whatever object one chooses.

(Dalai Lama 1994, p. 174)

Our own personality has a bearing on how easily we will slip into meditation. Some people realise a quieter atmosphere in their mind almost as soon as they begin to meditate. They have no difficulty watching their thoughts and observing their feelings. This is because some people are naturally very relaxed in themselves, and find that meditation simply enhances their inborn nature. Others have a lot going on in their lives and find it challenging to tame the mind. It can take them months and even years to glimpse a brief moment of clarity and emptiness.

Some people find being alone with their thoughts and feelings quite bewildering and unpleasant, and for a few people it is just too confronting. When a person's life is in turmoil and extremely stressful they often fill up all their time with 'outer' activities and don't allow themselves the time to think about what is actually happening because it's simply too painful.

Over the years of teaching I have found that it is not uncommon for someone to become very emotional and overwhelmed after a meditation. This is usually because it is the first time in years they have taken time out just for themselves. They often discover that the quietness and stillness within themselves is both extraordinary and beautiful. For others, it means coming to a grinding halt where they have the opportunity to look at their lives in a more detached way and maybe find some positive solutions and alternatives to their usual way of doing things.

Caution: Whatever your situation, always approach meditation slowly. If you become overwhelmed, simply open your eyes. Continue with the meditation when you are ready or, if you are having a lot of difficulty, practise under the supervision of an experienced teacher. Remember that the bigger the challenge, the greater the rewards are likely to be.

A life of only a single day spent in meditation, conjoined with wisdom, is better than living a hundred years unbalanced and confused.

(Dhammapad, in Choedak 1996)

Getting started

If meditation can be included easily into your daily routine you will be more likely to continue with the practice. Also, shorter sessions practised more often will prevent boredom and drowsiness and you will be more alert for the duration of the practice, rather than dozing off.

1. Choose a comfortable seated posture. Traditional postures are detailed in the chapter, 'Seated Postures for Pranayama & Meditation'. The posture, however, is less important than the meditation itself. So if you find the postures difficult, you may sit on a straight backed chair with your legs uncrossed and your feet on the ground, or on the floor with your legs to the front.

Always keep your spine as straight as possible. This ensures that your breathing continues to be smooth and even, the muscles of your back and abdomen remain relaxed and vital energy can flow easily up and down your spinal column. You can either sit with your buttocks on the floor or place one or two firm cushions under your tail bone. This will elevate your pelvis and tilt it slightly forward, which helps to relieve discomfort in your back. It is also acceptable to sit with your back against a wall for extra support.

2. Keep your eyes lightly closed. Some teachers recommend you leave your eyes open. I was taught to meditate with my eyes closed which is why I suggest this procedure, but the choice is yours.

3. Relax your arms from the shoulders and keep your elbows slightly bent. Rest your hands in one of the *mudras* detailed in the chapter of that name, or rest your palms down on your knees.

4. Hold your back straight but relaxed.

5. Tilt your chin slightly down. Press your lips lightly together and leave your teeth a little apart but make sure

132

The complete book of
yoga and meditation
for pregnancy

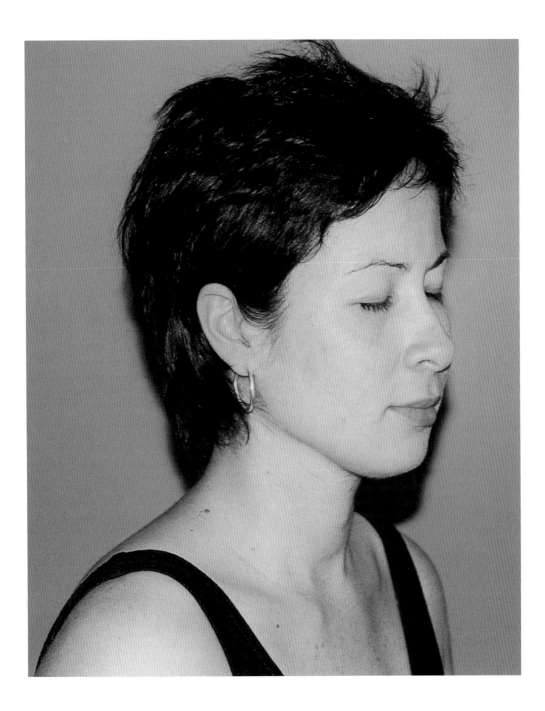

your mouth and jaw are relaxed.

6. Bring your attention to the position of your body. Notice any discomfort or tension in your body. Your body needs to be as relaxed as possible for successful meditation, so pay particular attention to releasing tension from those parts of your body before you begin.

7. When your body feels comfortable and relaxed, become conscious of your natural breath moving evenly in and out of your body. For the best results, I recommend 10 or 15 minutes of *pranayama* (breathing) before you begin your meditation. This will create a more relaxed body and a calmer state of mind.

8. Quieten the environment of your mind until you become still and centred. When you close your eyes to meditate you are alone with your thoughts and feelings and simply watching the activity in your mind.

9. When you feel you are still and relaxed, begin your meditation.

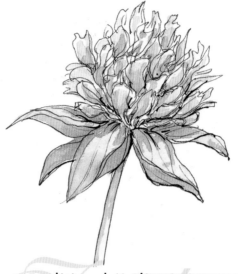

Traditional Meditations

1. Breath Awareness

Using Breath Awareness as a meditation is one of the purest and most consistently used practices. The breath is there with us every day of our lives and is therefore a logical point of focus. Sometimes it is more noticeable when we are exerting ourselves or during times of stress and anxiety. When we are relaxed and calm the resting breath is hardly noticeable at all. Whatever the circumstances, we breathe continually throughout our lifetime and for that reason meditation on the breath is one of the easiest to do and, for many people, the most gratifying. It is also a traditional practice that has been used by the ancient masters throughout time. A more detailed discussion of breath awareness can be found in the chapter, 'Pranayama'.

When time is spent following the natural breath, the mind becomes still

and the body automatically relaxes more deeply. Witnessing the breath quietly flowing in and out of the body as a form of meditation is a simple and effective way of turning the awareness inwards and observing the natural rhythms of the body, while it helps us to be clearly focused in each and every moment.

There are three aspects of a breath which can be followed for the purposes of this meditation.

(i) You can concentrate on the expansion and contraction of your chest as you breathe, becoming completely absorbed in the movements of your lungs.

(ii) You can observe the movement of your abdomen as you breathe. Your abdomen fills and your navel rises with each inhalation, and contracts with exhalation.

(iii) The breath in your nostrils can be felt, with the subtle differences of a cooler breath as you breathe in and

134

The complete book of
yoga and meditation
for pregnancy

the less obvious, warmer breath as you breathe out.

I suggest counting five breaths, with your awareness focused on the breath in your chest; then five breaths concentrating on the breath in your abdomen; followed by five more feeling the breath in your nostrils.

Each time you breathe in, feel you are drawing in all that is healing and balancing. When breathing out, dissolve and release all feelings and thoughts that are preventing you from being relaxed and still. With each breath be mindful of the whole breathing process.

As thoughts come into your mind, simply witness them in the same way you witness your breathing. In other words, watch yourself thinking and breathing just as you would watch the fish in the pond swimming into view and swimming out of view. It's as if there are two parts to you, the one who is breathing and thinking and the one who is watching yourself breathe and think.

When a thought arises, we must simply note that it has occurred, while at the same time remembering that it has come from nowhere, dwells nowhere, and goes nowhere, leaving no trace of its passage, just as a bird, in its course across the sky, leaves no mark of its flight. In this way, when thoughts arise, we can liberate them into the absolute expanse. When thoughts do not arise, we should rest in the open simplicity of the natural state.

(Khyentse 1994, p. 85)

The more time spent in the internal space of the mind watching yourself breathe, the more conscious you will also be of any thoughts that naturally come and go. When you continue to watch your thoughts, after some time you will notice there is a natural gap between one thought and

the next, where the mind is momentarily free of thoughts or suspended between one thought and another. The pause between thoughts sometimes feels eternal, endless and infinite and is the epitome of stillness. When we can hold our full awareness in this space, even for a brief moment, we witness a rare glimpse of pure awareness which is an experience of pure bliss. In yoga, this space is known as the *chitta kash*.

Counting breaths

Watching your breath is a valuable practice but the mind being what it is it will naturally roam, so it is quite normal to lose constant breath awareness. Counting your breaths is a useful way of controlling the wanderings of your mind and staying focused on your breathing. I like to count up to nine breaths, repeating up to that number for as long as I do the practice.

Counting backwards is also an excellent exercise for improving concentration as well as staying focused on your breathing. When you first do this you might find you lose count very easily. However, in time you will be able to watch your breath and count from a high number without losing concentration.

The Ujjayi Breath

The *Ujjayi* Breath – described in more detail in the chapter 'Pranayama' – can replace the natural breath as a point of focus during meditation. It has been described as the Breath of Tranquillity, the Psychic Breath and the Breath of the Mind because of the profound feelings experienced in the mind and ultimately in the body after even a short practice. The sound of the breath, the sensation of the breath at the throat and the

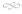

whole breathing process can be concentrated on. When you practise the *ujjayi* breathing as a meditation your whole attention becomes one pointed on the breath, where you consciously feel and hear yourself breathing in and out.

Sometimes in class I have seen people move very deeply into a quiet and peaceful place within themselves, when nothing else other than the *ujjayi* breathing is used as a meditation practice. It is an ideal exercise to use for finding that infinite space of the mind known as the *chitta kash*, and holding your awareness there. The longer the technique is done the slower you will breathe and the more centred and still you will become. In essence, you become one with the *ujjayi* breath.

You might like to begin this practice by blocking your ears and simply listening to the sound of the natural breath quietly moving in and out of the body. If you have ever been snorkelling or diving you will know what it's like to be in a still environment and have the sound of your breath as a constant companion. In a similar way when you spend time simply listening to the *ujjayi* breathing or the natural breath, your attention will naturally be drawn inwards as all other sounds will be less obvious, and it is the inner sound of the breath that is observed.

1. Focus on your natural breath and the sensation of air in your nostrils. Then move your attention to feeling the breath at the back of your throat and listening to the sound of your breathing. This is more profound when practised with your ears blocked.

2. When you are ready, unblock your ears. You can continue with the *ujjayi* breathing exercises by simply listening and feeling the effects of the practice, or by counting the breaths to

hold your attention more consistently in the present moment.

This exercise has been used by many women during labour as a way to stay calm and strong in themselves, especially when it is used in between contractions to recover from the last contraction and prepare for the next one.

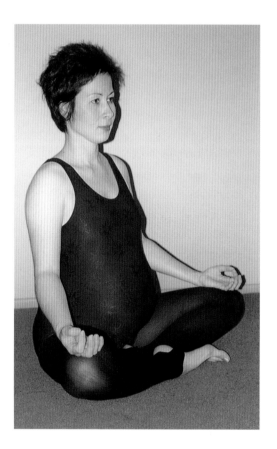

Opening and closing eyes

During meditation people relax so deeply that they sometimes drift off to sleep. This can be simply due to fatigue or a sense of 'letting go'. It can also be because the meditation is going on for too long, especially for beginners. I have found that if the eyes are opened and closed intermittently, falling asleep is less of a problem and the meditation can be maintained. In fact, some people have told me they were actually asleep when their eyes were closed but woke immediately when they were instructed to open their eyes.

136

The complete book of
yoga and meditation
for pregnancy

When this concept is combined with counting breaths it results in more control and awareness of your meditations. As your eyes are continuously opened and closed, the inner stillness experienced when your eyes are closed will also be felt when your eyes are open.

As a guideline, meditate on your breathing with your eyes closed for nine breaths, then with your eyes open for nine breaths. Repeat this as often as desired. The *ujjayi* breathing can be used here in place of your natural breath.

2. Body Awareness

It is an important point to remember that whatever you focus your attention on during meditation will probably become more intense. For example, if you concentrate on being calm then the feeling of calmness will increase. If you have your attention on how anxious you are feeling, then feelings of anxiety will increase, sometimes to the point where you have far less control over your behaviour and emotions. This is an especially important point to remember during labour.

The more conscious you can become of how you are feeling – physically and emotionally – the better you will be able to handle different or threatening situations especially when they take you completely by surprise. When we are more consciously aware of ourselves and have learnt how to be the observer and the witness we will more clearly know when we are relaxed or stressed by the way we are feeling and thinking

When we are relaxed our body looks and feels comfortable, our breathing is quiet and our thoughts are calm. However, in times of distress or shock, our body becomes tense, our stance defensive or protective, our breathing rapid and erratic and mentally we become disorientated and confused.

The next time you are relaxed and calm, spend a few minutes simply watching yourself. Be aware of your body, your thoughts and your breathing. Likewise, if you find yourself in a difficult situation, watch and learn from what you do, how you feel and how you react. This is a very simple and valuable exercise, and will help you to understand yourself more intimately. It is a life skill that will prove invaluable during your child-bearing years, and also later on in life.

The body awareness meditation can be done anywhere and at any time. It can be used as a brief exercise for becoming centred and mindful, or as a prelude to other meditation practices. It can also be the whole meditation practice, in itself, where you reflect on all aspects of your body. Your focus can be held on your face, for example, so that you really concentrate on all your different features as well as your face as a whole. You would then move your attention slowly to other parts of your body, observing them in an unattached manner but with full concentration.

When you are pregnant there are many changes occurring in your body as well as the movement of your baby in the womb to focus on. I feel this provides a valuable opportunity to spend time contemplating your pregnancy and observing the changes in your body while honouring yourself in all your womanly beauty during this time. It is also a wonderful opportunity to spend time connecting with your baby in the womb, noticing the movements increasing and changing as your baby develops and grows to maturity.

Often it is observing the little things about ourselves that has the most impact. These simple observations can make life really pleasant and enjoyable so that when something 'enormous' happens our awareness is finely tuned and we can experience the moment more consciously and with insight. Understanding body awareness is a valuable asset to use during labour as a way of 'bringing the mind home'. It will hold your attention in the present moment and help you to remain calm and centred while preparing for the next contraction. In the case of needing a caesarean delivery, it will enable you to be as relaxed as possible while you prepare for the procedure.

An excellent body awareness practice is to focus on your baby's movements, in contrast to the movements of your natural breath. Although the difference between the two is quite subtle, this exercise clearly distinguishes one movement from the other, and encourages a more specific and exacting concentration. From there, you can then concentrate on the contrast between these movements, and the feeling of complete stillness in the rest of your body. This is a valuable practice to do, as when you move your attention slowly from movement, to stillness, the distinction between the two becomes obvious.

3. Sound Awareness

Listening to different sounds can be a valuable form of contemplation and meditation. You can practise the Humming Breath and listen to your own unique, internal sound, or through 'om' chanting and sacred chanting. It can also be done by simply listening to the different sounds of nature.

The sounds of nature are always changing and incredibly varied, and using them as a meditation practice is purifying and uplifting. Sitting in a forest or in a park on a windy day where the trees are making a wide range of characteristic sounds can be quite energising, as is listening to the surf pounding on the shore or to a heavy rainfall. Then there are the softer sounds of nature which are more soothing and comforting to the senses, such as the gentle movements of a breeze in the trees, light rain, the sound of a stream, or birds communicating with each other in a forest.

Once you are fully involved with listening and can concentrate on simply observing sound, it's amazing what you become aware of and the variety of sounds you will hear around you. Remember, in meditation, whatever you focus your attention on increases. So, when you really listen and hear what is around you, you will realise there is an unlimited world of sounds to be explored and enjoyed. Imagine using your mind like a radar where you listen to the closer and louder sounds, then to the quieter sounds that are farther away.

Another practice is to listen to the sounds outside the room, and compare them to the sounds in the room. This is a particularly valuable technique for consciousness of the difference between the place where you are meditating and the outside environment. In many ways it's comparable to present moment awareness because when you are listening to the outer sounds it is similar to the thoughts being on the external. When you are consciously aware of the sounds inside the room or of your own breathing, your attention is directed towards the internal environment.

As you master the art of conscious listening, you will be able to extend your awareness far beyond what

138

The complete book of
yoga and meditation
for pregnancy

is audible and you will hear the silence that is beyond all sounds. In many ways, this is comparable to the infinite space of your mind. Then, as you bring your awareness back to what is around you, you will notice that the 'silence that is beyond the sounds' is also around you, within the room.

If you can meditate in a very quiet place, you will more easily observe the silence and stillness I refer to, to a point where you eventually immerse your whole awareness deeply into your self, to hear only the soft sound of your breath. When you become completely absorbed with hearing the gentle breath, the result is one of perfect quiet and serenity within your body and mind.

In this way you will discover the similarities between the peace, stillness and silence you perceive beyond sounds and that which you will discover deep within yourself. Ultimately, you bring the mind 'back home' to an atmosphere of complete calm.

4. The Gaze
(trataka)

The word *trataka* means to look or to gaze. This lovely yoga practice helps to improve concentration because where the eyes are directed the mind and thoughts will follow. It involves concentrating on a single stationary object. The Gaze is considered to be one of the most beneficial and easy to learn techniques, and will bring tranquillity and composure to even the most active mind.

You are free to choose any object you feel is easy to look at, but it needs to be something that won't create more ideas and thoughts in your mind. For example, you could use the face of a spiritual person, a religious symbol, an object you feel comfortable with or even a dot on the wall, as long as your focus

remains on the one object.

In my yoga and naturopathic practice, I often teach this technique to people who are stressed and in need of rest and relaxation, or who are unable to follow their breath because thoughts and worries flood their mind and prevent inner stillness. It is also simple to do at home or between classes or appointments. This is important because it gives us a sense of taking responsibility for their own health and wellbeing.

The candle meditation

In traditional yoga, the brightest point of a candle flame is used as the focal point. Most people discover this to be ideal because it is white, motionless and mesmerising.

For the purposes of pregnancy and labour, the candle meditation is one of the surest ways of establishing a quiet state of mind, and also of learning how to focus. This practice can be enjoyed easily at home. During labour, it can be used before going into hospital to help you relax and stay calm before the more active part of labour begins.

The candle meditation is also an excellent treatment for insomnia. A lady I know had been using sleeping pills for a number of years and decided to practise *tratak*a every night for 20 minutes before going to bed. She found after only a few days she no longer needed her sleeping pills, as the candle meditation gave her a deep and restful sleep. Physically, this practice will strengthen your eyes and stimulate your brain via the optic nerve, making *trataka* an ideal practice to do in conjunction with the Eye Exercises in the chapter, 'Warming up'.

1. For the best results, practise *trataka* at night in a darkened room. If you practise it during the day, make the

room as dark as possible. You will also be less distracted if your candle is in front of a blank wall. Many women love to practise *trataka* while relaxing in a warm bath perfumed with some of the relevant essential oils for pregnancy.

2. Place a lighted candle in front of you at least an arm's length from your face. Make sure the flame is at eye level and there are no breezes in the room. This helps keep the flame steady. This is

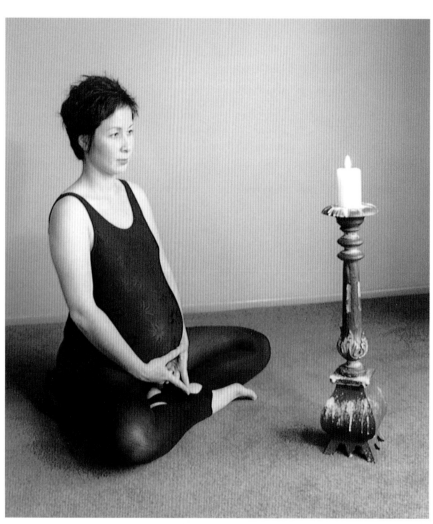

important because the idea of *trataka* is to become still, and if the flame is moving even slightly, your mind will be inclined to move too. Rest your hands on your legs in *chin, gyana, bhairava* or *yoni mudra*. Completely relax your body.

3. Close your eyes and bring your awareness to the position of your body,

your breathing and any thoughts that might come and go from your mind. As you clear the environment of your mind, begin to feel still and at peace. Remain with this feeling for a few minutes while breathing gently.

4. When you are ready, open your eyes and gaze at the brightest point of the flame. Blink if you need to. Close your eyes if you become aware of any eye discomfort. Sometimes the eyes can sting or water a little when you first practise *trataka*. Close your eyes before this happens.

5. After two or three minutes, close your eyes lightly. Keep your eyes closed for a short time as you observe your thoughts and your natural breath. Before you lose concentration, open your eyes and gaze at the flame again.

6. Repeat this procedure as often as desired. *Trataka* is generally practised for a minimum of 15 minutes, but this can be shortened or lengthened to suit your needs at the time. You will find the longer you spend gazing at the flame, the more centred and at peace you will become. After some time you might notice an 'internal' image of the flame between your eyebrows at the 'eyebrow centre'. You can meditate on the pure light of this internal image or you might like to visualise the light as a healing colour. This visualisation is detailed in the Candle Light meditation in the chapter, 'Visualisations & Creative Meditations'.

140

The complete book of
yoga and meditation
for pregnancy

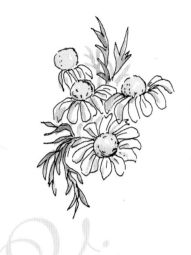

Visualisations and Creative Meditations

1. Colour meditations

All colours have their own unique healing qualities and they can be used in many different situations to assist in the healing process, to emphasise a particular feeling or to establish balance in the body and mind. They can enhance moods and affect the atmosphere of the mind and emotions, bringing about the right ambience for healing and change.

When colours are included in your meditations you might find they change from one colour to another even within the meditation. Quite often they are not the colours you would have chosen intellectually. Depending on how you feel on a particular day, you may wish to choose a colour that appeals to you, or you might prefer to allow a colour to spontaneously come into your mind. When you allow your intuition to do the choosing for you, you may be surprised by which colour comes to mind. It is important to trust your instincts and know that the colour in your mind is appropriate for you, rather than analysing why.

There has been extensive research done on the use of specific colours for particular problems and in different situations. However, sometimes it is best not to know too much about facts and details, as this could take your mind away from the inner stillness experienced during meditation. From this point of view I feel you are better to either choose a colour you are simply attracted to, or allow one to come to your mind in the quietness of the meditation. You will instinctively know the best colour for you on the day. However, if you are really drawn to one particular colour and are curious about the healing properties it has, the parts of the body it relates to or the emotions it balances, there are many interesting and informative books written on the subject of colour as a significant healing modality, available from most book shops today.

There are many ways to include colour into your meditations and I will explain a few techniques that can be used while you are pregnant and during labour.

Colour visualisation

1. Sit comfortably with your spine straight. Alternatively, you might like to do the colour meditation lying on the floor or in bed. Clear the environment of your mind and, if you are intending to do a long meditation, do some breathing exercises first to quieten your mind and relax your body.

2. When you are ready, bring to mind the qualities that you need to bring balance and harmony to your mind and body. If you are feeling fatigued this might be energy, if you are distressed or anxious it might be calmness, or maybe it is clarity if you can't stop thoughts flooding into you mind.

3. As you focus on what you need, bring to mind the colour that best represents the feeling you want to create. If you are unable to visualise a colour, then just think about it as if you were daydreaming.

4. Your chosen colour can be seen as a soft mist or vapour all around your body completely surrounding you, or alternatively you might see it as a cloak or another type of covering over your body. How you see it is completely up to you. The colour can be quite vivid and bright, or of softer more subtle tones, and it might be very close to your body or filling the room where you are meditating.

5. The colour can be enclosed in a shimmering silver or gold bubble to hold in the healing vibrations. Visualising a colour inside a bubble

makes you feel safe and secure, and means the healing qualities of the colour do not disperse into the atmosphere. The bubble can also act as an imaginary filter that allows goodness and healing to come into the bubble while deflecting any unwanted influences.

6. This is a popular meditation to do during labour. The colour can be seen around you, or filling the room where you are having the baby. In this way all those who are there with you will benefit from your potent meditation. You might visualise a colour deep inside your womb surrounding your baby, a colour that is filled with feelings of love and welcome.

When you are in labour a colour can be visualised inside the birth canal where you imagine your baby moving easily and gently. A beautiful colour can then be imagined around the cervix, as you visualise it slowly and gradually opening for the easy delivery of your baby. These visualisations will mentally assist with the birthing process, and when your baby is born visualise a beautiful colour completely surrounding you, your new baby and your partner.

The rainbow

The colours of the *chakras* are said by many authorities to be the same as those of the rainbow. There are, however, some teachings which suggest the colours are the same up to the heart *chakra*, but from there on they are not the same colours as those of a rainbow. Personally, I feel that when the colours of the rainbow are used for this meditation we are working in harmony with one of nature's most glorious phenomena. It really gets down to the feeling experienced in the meditation, and if the rainbow colours feel right for you, then they are appropriate.

This meditation flows naturally

142

The complete book of
yoga and meditation
for pregnancy

from the Pyramid meditation which is described later in this chapter.

1. Visualise you are seated inside a perfectly balanced pyramid. Sometimes, I also begin by suggesting that you are in a beautiful, open place in nature that feels both empowering and peaceful. This will often create a feeling of space and allow you to make your pyramid as large as you want instead of thinking it has to fit into the room where you are meditating. Choose a place that is a potent symbol for you and one that has a limitless feeling to it.

2. When you have the outline of the pyramid in your mind, visualise the first colour of the rainbow, which is red. Imagine that the pyramid and everything inside is brilliant red, and that the colour is completely surrounding your whole body. Hold that image in your mind as you breathe easily and gently, absorbing the colour and the vibrations of that colour into your body and mind. Remain with the colour red for as long as you wish to.

3. Visualise the colour orange. Feel the colour orange all around you, noticing any differences within yourself when you change colour. Breathe the colour orange deeply into your whole being.

4. In your own time, imagine the colour has changed from orange to yellow, brilliant and glowing all around you. Again, hold this in your mind for as long as you wish to.

5. The next colour is green and as you visualise yourself inside a green pyramid be aware of the differences you are feeling with the new colour all around you.

6. Next, the colour changes from green to blue, a beautiful midday blue. Breathe this healing colour into every cell in your body, your mind and into your womb to surround your baby. As you continue with the meditation, be very conscious of the colours you are the most akin with and the different feelings that they each have.

7. From blue, the colour becomes indigo. Hold in your mind the image of yourself seated inside a pyramid, glowing like the most beautiful blue sapphire you can imagine.

8. The last colour of the rainbow is purple. See the indigo merging in with the magnificent purple. Again hold this in your mind and feel the stillness in your body and the clearness in your mind for as long as you wish to.

9. When the rainbow colours are complete, I then like to imagine that the pyramid becomes radiant gold: the frame, the outline, the walls and the whole interior. This meditation can take as little as 10 minutes, but you might become totally engrossed in the colours and the feelings you are experiencing and find it has taken half an hour or more. Visualising the colours of the rainbow, in whatever format appeals to you the most, is a beautiful way to meditate and has always been well liked in my classes. The healing properties of the individual colours will be felt immediately to give you balance, harmony and a great inner strength.

The candle light

This meditation follows naturally on from the candle meditation (trataka). When you have been practising trataka for 15 or 20 minutes you might begin to feel the image of the light remaining at the point between your eyebrows, even when your eyes are closed. You may then extend the meditation and visualise the light from the flame becoming a healing colour.

1. Imagine the light of the flame filling your whole body and taking on the shape of your silhouette. When you

Meditations
Visualisations
and creative meditations

do this, you might like to visualise the light as a particular colour. The colour could be slightly varied in different parts of your body. You will eventually have an image of yourself as a body of light or colour, or a feeling of being filled with light.

2. The light can also be seen in your womb, as if you have turned on a switch and are able to see your baby in the womb. You may imagine the light – or colour – completely surrounding your baby. With this beautiful image in your mind, you and your baby can spend some quiet moments together with thoughts and feelings of love and welcome.

3. The light can be imagined around the outside of your body. You may wish to visualise the light quite close to your body, or see yourself as very small inside a vast expanse of radiant light. Your vision of light can then be held inside a shimmering bubble which is there to hold the light and the feeling all around you. Many women have enjoyed this practice because it gives a warm and gentle feeling and can be used to enhance serenity, calmness and a sense of safety.

4. To combine all three variations, see yourself and your womb filled with a brilliant light or colour, and this whole image completely surrounded by light and encased in a beautiful bubble.

2. Spinal column meditations

Using awareness of the spinal column as a form of meditation is one of the best practices for centring concentration and consolidating a focused awareness. It can be approached in a number of different ways from simple breath awareness up and down your spine, to more elaborate visualisations incorporating colour, etc.

I will discuss how it is basically practised, as well as a few variations that have proven both inspiring and effective for my students.

Breath, light and colour

1. Before you begin the meditation spend some time quietening your mind and becoming still, using the Breath Balancing posture with either the natural breath or the *ujjayi pranayama*. I suggest you then practise one or two of the breathing exercises for about 10 minutes to increase your concentration and attention on the breath.

2. When you are ready, direct your awareness and your breath to your spinal column in the centre of your body. Feel your breath within your spinal column and, as you breathe in, move your awareness from the base of your spine to the top of your head. As you breathe out, move your awareness down your spine to your tail bone.

3. Continue with this practice, feeling the breath and *prana* moving up and down your spine. You will become very conscious of your inner self and notice a feeling of steadiness and strength in your position.

4. A visualisation can also be included by imagining light or colour within your spinal column, moving up and down with your breath.

Earth and sky

This is a very balancing practice for the mind and the body as it gives a feeling of being grounded, focused and secure within yourself. You simply concentrate on the symbolic influence of the earth below you and the sky above you.

1. As you breathe in, feel the energy from the earth being drawn up into your body to establish balance and harmony in your physical self. When

144

The complete book of
yoga and meditation
for pregnancy

you breathe out, imagine you are drawing clarity, knowledge and wisdom into yourself from the unlimited expanse of sky above you. When this is done, the earth can be seen as a symbolic reflection of our physical self, while the sky represents the more divine and spiritual aspects of our natures, in other words connecting the physical and the spiritual through the visualisation. Many people find this meditation very grounding and stabilising for the mind and the body.

2. Colour can also be added to this visualisation. Simply imagine a colour coming up into your body from deep in the earth. As it passes from the earth through your body it might change from a deep earthy tone to a lighter colour as it moves up into your body. When you take your awareness up to the sun, draw on the sun's radiant colour and bring it down into your body while breathing out.

Be as creative as you want with the visualisation of colour. Get in touch with establishing physical balance and wellbeing from the earth, and spiritual awareness and harmony from the symbolic sun. It is interesting to note which colour you see at the centre of your body where the two energies meet. I feel it represents a balance of the physical and the spiritual aspects of your self. Quiet reflection on this colour

could be valuable as a meditation practice if you are needing to establish and maintain balance within your self, either during times of stress or even when you are in labour.

3. The tree meditations
A tree is 'the embodiment of life, the point of union of the three realms, heaven, earth and water.'

(Fontana 1993, p. 100)

I first discovered the Tree meditation in Phyllis Krystal's book, *Cutting the Ties that Bind* (1989), and I have found it to be both beneficial and well liked in all my classes. Trees are incredibly beautiful, diverse and unique. They give us constant beauty. Trees have always been considered a special treasure to humans as they provide a source of food and shelter; wood for tools, weapons, houses, boats, transport; fuel, and medicines from their roots, bark, leaves and berries. They also provide shelter and food for insects, reptiles, animals and birds. Most significantly, without trees our planet and all living things would die. The tree has been a symbol of life in many cultures, and the Buddha became enlightened sitting under a Bodhi tree in India.

In ancient times trees were objects of worship by the druids and ordinary people all over the world. In some middle eastern countries,

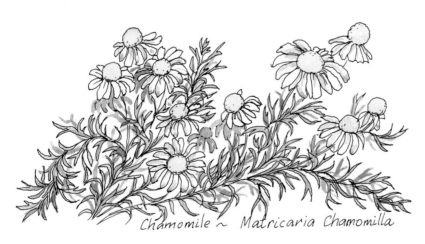

Chamomile ~ Matricaria Chamomilla

apparently, there were 'sacred groves in which to practise phyllomancy, the art of divination by listening to the rustling of leaves.' (Walker 1995, p. 202) What a lovely thought for a meditation practice!

The evergreen tree represents a healthy life, abundance and prosperity, while the deciduous tree represents the cycle of life corresponding to the seasons and the cycle of birth, life, death and rebirth. In summer, a tree is full and lush with abundant growth made possible by the warmth and light of the summer sun. In autumn, the leaves change and die as the days become cooler and there is less light. Winter is a time for inner growth, regeneration and preparation for rebirth of the tree's energy, followed by new growth and signs of new life in the spring.

The tree is a potent symbol of strength, stability, nurturing and grace. Some women feel unsure of their ability to cope during labour or as a mother. Others might not be feeling completely happy about the changes in their pregnant bodies and seem to have lost their usual self-confidence and joy of life. This practice provides a feeling of inner strength and quiet confidence to help women cope with the many changes, fears and doubts that often surface as pregnancy progresses. It is also invaluable after the birth when everything is new and often overwhelming.

In this meditation the tree is seen to stand strong between heaven and earth. The earth is conceived of as the mother symbol, representing the more physical aspects of our selves. The sun is visualised as the father symbol, relating more to our spiritual aspects. It can be practised in your usual place for meditation or, for a more realistic feel, you might like to sit against a tree in a

forest or in your own garden. The Tree meditation can be practised as three separate meditations or as a continuous flow from one exercise to the next.

The nurtured tree

1. Spend a little time preparing for the meditation by quietening your mind and becoming still. When you are relaxed and centred, visualise yourself standing before a fully grown, healthy tree. This might be a familiar tree, one you have seen in a photo or an imaginary tree with magical qualities.

2. Visualise the tree in all its beauty standing firmly in the ground. Visualise the height of the tree, the colour of the trunk, the branches and the leaves. Imagine the earth below the tree and the sun shining directly above it giving light and warmth to the leaves and to the earth.

3. When you are ready, go over to the tree and lean against it with your arms outstretched, feeling how easily the tree takes your weight and supports you. Then sit on the ground with your spine against the trunk, feeling safe and secure.

4. Bring your attention to the earth beneath you and visualise the roots of the tree spreading far into the earth holding the tree firmly in the ground. Imagine the roots seeking nutrients deep in the earth. Know that the earth has provided all that the tree has needed, from the time it was a seed, then a tiny seedling, to its full height as you see it in your meditation.

5. As you breathe in, feel you are drawing into yourself the earth's energies. These are the energies of the symbolic mother providing you with the love, tenderness, reassurance and strength you need to help you feel strong and secure within yourself. As you breathe out, release all doubts and

insecurities from within yourself.

6. Now visualise the sun above the tree and feel the warmth of the sun's rays. Imagine the sunlight shining on the leaves and branches. In your mind, be aware that the sun has provided the tree with the light and warmth to grow tall and strong, ever since it was a tiny seed in the ground.

7. As you breathe in, imagine you are drawing energy from the sun, feeling the warmth giving you life. Think of all the qualities a father gives a child so that it can grow wise and strong. Qualities such as confidence, courage, inner strength, knowledge and wisdom. Feel you are drawing them into yourself with each breath. As you breathe out, release all uncertainty.

8. Continue to do this practice for as long as you wish to, before simply reflecting on the qualities you have brought into yourself through the meditation.

Releasing and regeneration

1. Imagine you are the tree. Visualise yourself standing firm and secure in the ground, filled with confidence and inner strength.

2. Although you feel very strong, you might also be aware of some unwanted feelings that have been either holding you back in some way or have prevented you from maintaining feelings of strength and confidence in your daily life. Imagine that these limiting ways of thinking and feeling are leaves falling to the ground. All your unresolved fears, doubts and negative beliefs are no longer attached to you but are falling away from you as dead leaves.

Sometimes all the leaves will fall

to the ground, while in other meditations you might only see a few falling, suggesting that you either have only a little to release at that time, or that it is appropriate to do the meditation in gradual stages of release rather than all at once. It is best to go with the images that come up for you in the meditation rather than trying to force anything, trusting instead that your intuitive nature knows what is best in that moment.

3. These old leaves are then replaced with new growth. Visualise

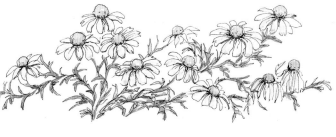

buds, leaves and flowers to show new ways of thinking, more positive thoughts and a fresh life within you. Be as creative as you want to be and spend as long as you need to so you are able to not only imagine it in your mind but also feel it in your heart.

Four seasons

1. This time, see the tree changing as it moves through the four seasons.

2. When the meditation is complete you might then like to illustrate it, showing all the significant changes. This will bring the meditation from your conscious mind into the physical realm. For example, the first tree is a beautiful summer tree full of leaves and with the sun above it. Feel the warmth of the summer sun and spend some time visualising the tree in all its summer glory. The second tree represents a tree in autumn, where the leaves are changing colour and falling to

Meditations
Visualisations
and creative meditations

the ground, symbolising the release of outmoded ideas and beliefs in preparation for change. When you meditate on the autumn tree feel that the sun has less light and warmth than in the summer, and that although the leaves are falling to the ground they are also acting to replenish the earth and ultimately give benefit to the tree. The third is a tree in winter, maybe with snow on the ground. The sun has the least warmth and light of any of the seasons. Imagine the tree is standing bare but inwardly it is doing all the growth and healing in preparation for regeneration and rebirth in the spring. The fourth is the tree in spring, abundant with new growth such as beautiful flowers and fruit. Even imagine animals living in the tree to represent fulfillment and joy.

3. You might like to complete your illustrated meditation by visualising and then drawing another summer tree. This time the tree has even more beauty, grace and strength than the first tree because any doubts, unwanted feelings and beliefs are now replaced with abundant new growth.

Note: It is important not to get caught up in how well you draw. Your drawings can be quite simple because the importance lies in acknowledging what you have visualised and illustrating those concepts. When you meditate in this very creative way and use some simple illustrations to express your feelings, you will realise the power of your mind when it is utilised in a positive and imaginative way.

The wish fulfilling tree

When I first introduced this meditation to my classes, I was really surprised at how much the women enjoyed and appreciated it. The women told me that it encouraged them to have real goals about their pregnancies and birth, and about becoming a mother. It gave them the opportunity to explore how they felt, and what they really wanted at this special time in their lives. I suggested they actually draw their magical tree, as I have suggested in the four seasons visualisation, so as to bring their visualisation from the meditative states of the inner mind into the conscious world.

1. The wish fulfilling tree can be a regular tree in your garden or in a forest, which you are quite familiar with. However, as this particular tree has magical qualities and will carry your dreams and wishes, you might like to imagine it as something a little ethereal or celestial, not quite of this world.

2. In your mind see the tree standing majestic and strong, being aware of its size, shape, type of leaves, and surroundings. You can imagine brilliant sunshine giving light and warmth to your tree, or maybe gentle moonlight making your tree glow, luminous and soft.

3. Imagine you are either leaning up against your tree or gazing at it from a distance. Take a moment or two to relax and stay with these thoughts and feelings, knowing this is your own special tree.

4. Make a wish concerning your pregnancy and visualise it on the tree either as a coloured ball or a beautiful coloured light. Use your imagination. Then, make another wish about your labour, about the birth, and another about your first moments together with your baby. Make a wish about being a mother in the early weeks of your baby's life, and then when your baby is crawling, takes those first steps, and is one year old. Be as creative as you want and place as many wishes on the tree as you desire.

148

The complete book of
yoga and meditation
for pregnancy

∞

This can be repeated as often as you like, sometimes making only one or two wishes, while at other times filling the whole tree with your fondest dreams. Look at your wish fulfilling tree and see all your goals and desires in their symbolic form. Hold this in your mind for as long as you can.

4. The Mountain

Sit, then, as if you were a mountain, with all the unshakable, steadfast majesty of a mountain.
(Sogyal Rinpoche 1994a, p. 35)

I have found when I use the image of a mountain for the purpose of meditation that most people relate to it easily and receive excellent results. Mountains have always been symbols of great power, indomitable energy and enormous beauty and possess an almost godlike presence. Man has been fascinated by their seemingly invincible force. We are in awe of their beauty and incredible atmosphere. Being in the mountains can be a dynamic experience, as the elements are sometimes at their most volatile and fervent, while at other times it can be so still that the silence is 'deafening'.

Mountains have been chosen as places for retreats where masters of meditation and devout yogis spend many years in uninterrupted solitude. Monasteries, temples, shrines and other religious monuments have been constructed high in the mountains. The higher the mountain, the closer are the heavenly realms and the deities of worship.

Mountains have been said to be the meeting places of heaven and earth, as the base of the mountain is on the earth and relates to our physical reality while the top of the mountain is reaching towards heaven and represents our spiritual natures.

One of the oldest deities in India was Chomo-Lung-Ma, 'Goddess Mother of the Universe', whose mountain shrine is now known to Westerners by a man's name, Everest. Still feminine, however, is the Himalayan peak Annapurna, meaning 'Great Breast Full of Nourishment'
(Walker 1995).

1. When the seated body is seen in silhouette it resembles the shape of a mountain, wide at the base and tapering into a peak at the top of the head. This image will make you feel extremely still, steady, solid and immovable.

2. See all your unwanted thoughts swirling around your head, in the same way that wind, snow and sleet rage around the top of a mountain. Like a mountain you are not disturbed or moved by all this mental activity, no matter how strong the distraction or how severe the storm.

3. See the wind decreasing as your thoughts subside. See the sun shining brilliantly in an azure sky, bringing clarity, light and illumination to your mind. Alternatively, you might imagine that it is midnight, the sky is like black velvet filled with stars and there is a brilliant full moon shimmering over the mountain, bringing enrichment and clearness to your thoughts.

5. The Golden Spiral

The Golden Spiral is similar to the Mountain meditation in that you are sitting in the shape of an inverted 'V', so that your form is wide at the base and comes to a peak. When this spiral is visualised it seems to lift your awareness upwards and you will feel more present in your mind than in your body. I have watched people doing this practice and they actually sit taller and lift their heads higher as the spiral formation is imagined.

I have chosen the colour gold because it is often said to be the colour that most expresses divine principles and it is the colour that symbolises majesty, wisdom and purity. It is also the colour of the sun which gives light and warmth. In Hindu mythology, the colour of gold represents truth. The ancient Egyptians connected it to the sun god Ra who, for them, all life was dependent upon. In the story of Jason and the Golden Fleece, gold stood for immortality and was found on the tree of life. Many ancient cultures felt that gold has the qualities of the Sun, in that it always remains untarnished.

1. Begin by sitting on the floor in a cross-legged position. If you are not comfortable in a cross-legged position, do this particular meditation in a chair so that you are able to still visualise the golden spiral all around you. Spend a little time becoming quiet and still.

2. When you are ready visualise you are inside a golden circle which can be as large or small as you like. This is a very centring practice and helps to hold the awareness within that space. The circle represents unbroken energy because it lacks a beginning and an end and it is often considered to be perfect and eternal. It is a feminine symbol and a protective symbol, often associated with equality and balance (Walker 1995, p. 14). It is interesting to note that, in our culture, a gold wedding band represents unbroken love.

3. From the circle, slowly draw the gold upwards so that it begins to form a spiral gradually moving up and around your body. The 'ancients believed that energy, physical and spiritual, flowed in spiral form.' (Fontana 1993, p. 75) Walker also mentions that 'the spiral was connected with the idea of death and rebirth; entering the mysterious earth womb,

penetrating to its core, and passing out again by the same route.' (Walker 1995, p. 14) The spiral will become narrower the higher up your body it goes until it reaches a peak above the centre of your head.

4. Imagine that the space inside the spiral is filled with complete balance, harmony and wellbeing on all levels and is of the purest, most peaceful energy. Hold this in your mind as you breathe quietly and gently.

5. When you want to come out of the meditation slowly reverse the spiral formation until you again visualise you are sitting inside a golden circle.

6. The Pyramid

The Pyramid, like the Golden Spiral and the Mountain, is used for becoming centred and still. If you are the type of person who likes symmetrical and equally proportioned structures rather than circles, you might gain more from the Pyramid meditation than from the Golden Spiral.

Each of these visualisations very quickly deepens your level of concentration and develops a one pointed awareness and can be used as a meditation practice by itself, or as part of a more in-depth meditation.

A pyramid is perfectly balanced with all proportions of equal dimensions. Pyramids are 'the most evocative of three dimensional symbols … Its apex symbolises the highest point of spiritual attainment, with the body of the structure representing man's ascent through the hierarchy of enlightenment.' (Fontana 1993, p. 59) When you visualise yourself inside a pyramid, you will notice increased feelings of strength, stability, security and balance. When colour is included the benefits are enhanced considerably.

150

The complete book of
yoga and meditation
for pregnancy

1. Prepare for the meditation by sitting comfortably with your spine straight and your body relaxed. When you are ready, visualise you are sitting in the centre of a large square. This outline might be seen as light or a particular colour.

2. From each corner of the square draw four lines of equal height that meet at a central point above your head. The pyramid can be as large as you like. The walls of the pyramid can be solid or they might appear as clear or coloured glass.

3. When the pyramid is complete, hold the image in your mind as you follow your natural breath. You can use the natural breath or you might prefer to use the *ujjayi pranayama*. Any of the other breathing techniques can also be used.

4. You may like to visualise a particular colour inside the pyramid using the directions for Colour meditation earlier in this chapter, as a guide. In particular, the Rainbow meditation follows on very naturally from the Pyramid.

5. Breathe in the qualities of the colour and of the pyramid with each breath. Continue to do this for as long as you wish. You will notice the effects are quite inspiring. This is an ideal practice to do if you don't have a lot of time but need to feel the results fairly quickly.

6. You might like to visualise the sun above the pyramid. Imagine its warmth and light streaming into the top, filling the pyramid with light and warmth. Alternatively, you can imagine that the sun is a golden ball of vital energy and purity above the apex of the pyramid, from where a golden rain falls continuously to completely fill the pyramid. Be as creative as you want to be and use any of these suggestions to open the way for your own visualisations and creative meditations.

7. The Ocean of Abundance

I would like to include here a very special visualisation technique which comes from Phyllis Krystal's wonderful book, *Cutting the Ties that Bind* (1989, p. 164). She calls it 'The Wave for Relaxation'. I have often included it in my classes and many people have commented on the effectiveness of combining this visualisation with deep breathing for overcoming stress and tension.

In this meditation, a slow healing wave of water brings peace, balance and harmony to every aspect of yourself, and takes away with it all physical, emotional and mental stress.

This is ideal to do when you are having trouble sleeping, or when you are bothered by too many unwanted thoughts or uncomfortable feelings. It is also ideal for labour, to assist in establishing quietness and clamness between contractions. For example, imagine any physical tension, anxiety, fear or restlessness being washed away from you as you breathe out leaving you centred and calm as you prepare for the next contraction with a gentle and peaceful outlook.

1. Begin by lying on the floor with your body relaxed and your eyes lightly closed. Imagine you are lying on a beach at the water's edge. The ocean is a symbol of abundance, the salt in the water is the universal cleanser and healer

and the colour of the ocean is very healing, nurturing and calming.

2. As you breathe in deeply, imagine a wave moving slowly over your body, either to your throat or right over your face, bringing healing and peace to all aspects of your being.

3. When you breathe out, imagine the wave moving back down over your body and out into the ocean, leaving you cleansed and soothed. Visualise all discomfort, tension and imbalance in your physical body being removed, all unwanted thoughts and confusion being released from your mind, and any negative emotions such as fear, grief, anger or anxiety being released and washed away.

4. Repeat this as many times as you feel is appropriate, with each breath feeling and sensing yourself becoming lighter and more relaxed on all levels.

8. The Sultana

A couple of years ago I went to a Stewart Wilde seminar where he presented the Sultana meditation as part of his program, to encourage clarity of mind and to increase deep concentration. Although this is definitely not a traditional yoga practice, I am including it here because it is an excellent practice for complete beginners to meditation and for those who find it difficult to stay focused as it teaches the concepts of one pointed awareness and contemplation.

The sultana meditation takes between 10 and 15 minutes, and the majority of people find they are able to stay completely absorbed in the practice without being distracted. This is quite an achievement as under normal circumstances the attention span for most people is no more than two minutes before the mind becomes preoccupied by passing thoughts. When I introduce this practice everyone is totally amazed by where the time has gone and how incredible it is to concentrate so deeply on a single sultana for 15 minutes. It certainly puts a whole new meaning on eating and on the sense of taste.

1. Sit in a position that will be comfortable for at least 15 minutes. Have your eyes lightly closed. Place a sultana in the palm of your hand. Become aware of its lightness, yet also its ever increasing pressure and the surprising weight that a single sultana can have.

2. After some time, place the sultana in your mouth. Explore its contours, texture, shape and size for as long as you wish. When you are ready, slowly chew the sultana. Experience the explosion of sweetness on your tastebuds. Finally, swallow the sultana.

3. Allow as much time as you need to do this and be as detached as possible from watching how long it takes. When the sultana is finally swallowed you will be aware of the sweet aftertaste which you can remain focused on until you are ready to come out of the meditation.

Echinacea augustifolia

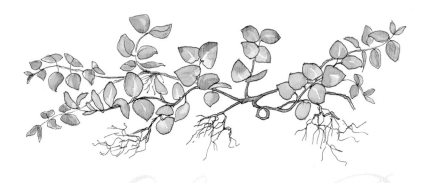

Your Baby & Yourself

These three meditations are without doubt the most important for this book as they focus on your baby in the womb, your pregnancy, the miracle of birth and the wonder of being a woman.

1. Your baby

This first meditation is an important practice as many women find it difficult to actually connect with the baby growing and developing in their womb, or to accept it as their own child and a real person. Visualising your baby in the womb enables you to imagine what your baby might look like and to spend time with your child before the birth. Even if you cannot create a clear picture in your mind, by spending time thinking about your baby your feelings will begin to flow and the remarkable union of mother and child will start to take place. During the nine months of your pregnancy this meditation will help you to stay focused on what is

actually happening in your body, and to contemplate the absolute miracle of pregnancy. It will also allow you the time to appreciate how extraordinary life is.

This quiet meditation will give you some precious moments alone together, where gentle thoughts and feelings of love and welcome can be shared with your baby. For some women, the idea of having conversations with this 'unknown' in their womb might seem a little unconventional and a bit strange. However, with a little time and especially as the pregnancy progresses, you will feel more comfortable with this notion and look forward to the quiet times together before the birth.

It is especially valuable if you were unaware of your pregnancy and feel you missed out on the early months, or if you were too unwell to think about the fact that there is a living person in your womb. Some women feel they are deprived of time if their baby is born early and they missed the last weeks of pregnancy and preparation for the birth.

It is also significant after the birth if the labour was difficult and your energy was taken up with recovering your strength, or if there were complications and problems after delivery which prevented you from spending the early days together. In all these situations, much of the 'getting to know you' and bonding has occurred before the birth through inner reflection and quiet meditation, so that you are connected to your baby no matter what happens before or after the birth.

1. When you are visualising your baby in the womb you can imagine all the delicate features, the shape of the head, the eyes and the eyebrows, the tiny nose and nostrils and other features of your baby's face. You can imagine the curved shape of the back and the legs tucked up in the fetal position, the little toes and even the tiny toe nails. The arms are folded and you can visualise the hands, the little fingers and the fingernails. See the umbilical cord floating in the waters of the womb connected to a healthy placenta, supplying your baby with all that it needs to grow strong and, as you feel your baby moving, imagine these movements in your mind. Spend as much time as you wish pondering the wonder of life and your baby in the womb.

2. Colour can be used during this meditation and it is something many women easily relate to. The colour can be seen inside the womb as a soft mist or vapour, or maybe a strong image of colour will be present. The colour is

The complete book of
yoga and meditation
for pregnancy

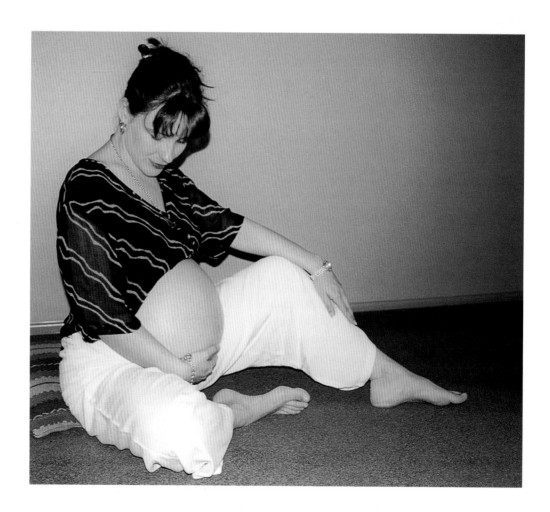

always one that represents the feelings of love and welcome you are wanting to express to the baby, and remember to be as creative as you want to be, as this is a very special and unique time in your life that will be over before you even realise.

3. When your baby is born, remember to make some extra time away from the usual activities of day-to-day life for you to simply be with each other. This could be giving your baby a gentle massage after a bath, having a warm bubble bath together, making sure the answer phone is turned on while you are feeding or playing together so you won't be disturbed, or simply indulge yourself by sitting quietly for a few minutes and watching your baby sleep. You will discover how quickly your baby changes and grows, almost before your eyes, and as you have made the time to be alone together during pregnancy, do the same thing as often as you can after the birth.

2. Embracing your baby

During pregnancy, it is sometimes hard to fully realise that at the end of the nine months you will have your baby in your arms and that you will be at the beginning of a very new and remarkable journey. There are so many changes to cope with that to actually imagine seeing your baby for the first time, can be lost in all the other information.

I feel it is very important to visualise beyond pregnancy and labour and to prepare for those first precious moments together using this creative and intimate meditation. Even though you will be planning ahead throughout the pregnancy preparing a nursery, buying clothes and other necessities for your new baby, it is unusual to take the time out to visualise the first time you will hold your baby in your arms and

look into each other's eyes. This meditation seems to bring the reality of what will happen after pregnancy into focus while it gives women the opportunity to visualise themselves as a mother with a new baby.

1. I feel it is best to concentrate on the actual place where you are planning to deliver because this will create a more realistic atmosphere in the meditation.

2. Become relaxed and still, following the flow of your natural breath quietly moving in and out of your body. Clear the environment of your mind of all other thoughts and when you are ready, imagine you are in the place you have chosen for the birth.

3. In the delivery room with you are all those people you have asked to be there for the birth of your baby, including your partner, the doctor and midwife and others you might have asked. Feel safe, secure and completely supported by these people knowing they are all there to assist you and your baby through the birthing process. Imagine the atmosphere of the room is calm, quiet and peaceful and feel very comfortable in this place.

4. You might like to imagine a beautiful colour filling the room, surrounding all who are there, bringing feelings of love, joy and welcome.

5. Now visualise your newborn baby resting in your arms for the first time. Feel the weight of your baby in your arms. See your baby's face and features, observe the tiny movements it is making with its mouth and eyes, look at its beautiful little fingers and hear the new sounds and the breathing. Touch your baby's skin and feel how soft and smooth it is. As you absorb all these images and feelings as you look into your baby's eyes and simply love each other. Hold these mental pictures in

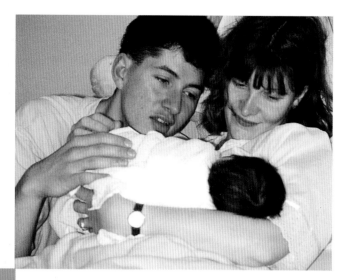

your mind acknowledging the absolute wonder of the moment.

6. In your visualisation you might like to include your partner and others who are special to you and your baby, feeling they are there to love and welcome your baby into the world. A beautiful colour or light can also be seen all around you and your baby, illuminating the image and enhancing the feelings you most want to create.

3. Honouring yourself

This very special meditation is, in many ways, a summary of what this book is all about – honouring yourself as a woman during your pregnancy.

Honouring yourself as a woman is a meditation that really needs to be at the very beginning of the book, as well as here towards the end, so you are constantly reminded through all the days of your pregnancy of how precious this time is in your life and how fortunate you are to be born a woman.

Your journey through pregnancy is such a brief moment in a lifetime, that it is often over before you have the opportunity to really become absorbed in all that has occurred. While you are pregnant and going through the many changes in your body, as well as coping with morning sickness, the loss of your

waist, increased weight and cellulite, fluid retention, fatigue, headaches and all the other ailments that so often accompany pregnancy, you can easily miss the beauty of the transformation and the absolute radiance that all pregnant women exhibit. Women are often at their loveliest and most luminous during pregnancy.

I feel it is important to reflect on these rare moments – brief as they are – and allow yourself the luxury of feeling warm and at peace with the miracle of what is happening to you. It is also important to acknowledge that your life is in a moment of transition between one aspect of being a woman and another. The idea of becoming a mother is such an awesome thought filled with so many varied emotions including wonder, fear, anxiety and a completely different kind of love, a love you will recognise the moment your baby is born, or even earlier during your pregnancy.

Pregnancy is a creative time that in no way overlooks the joy of simply being a woman, but instead is another phase of the feminine nature, where you acknowledge and appreciate yourself as a pregnant woman approaching motherhood.

This does not need to be a formal meditation, but instead just some time away from the usual activities of your day where you can be alone with your thoughts and feelings about being a pregnant woman. These private moments can help you come to terms with the many changes occurring in your body, in your day to day living and within all your relationships, while reflecting on the miracle of life itself. This inner reflection will also help you to appreciate that your life will never really be the same once your baby is born – but it will be enriched beyond

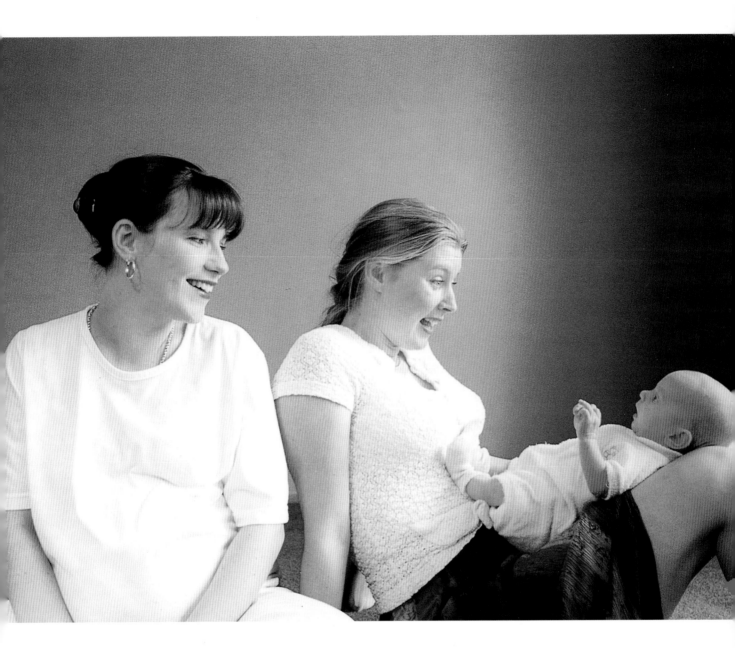

words for the rest of your life.

Meditation of this type will keep you more 'present' in your pregnancy and help you to hold the essence of what it really means. After your child is born, and later takes those first magical steps into a whole new world, is waving goodbye to you on the first day of school, or is taller than you and has pubic hair – then will you appreciate the time you spent in quiet reflection during your pregnancy. When these events happen you will realise how quickly time has gone and a little inner reflection during pregnancy somehow alleviates the well hidden, secret melancholia, mixed with joy and wonder, that women often feel when they look at their grown children.

A little time during pregnancy spent honouring yourself as a woman will connect you with your inherent feminine wisdom and the miracle of life. It will also act as a reminder for you to continue to take some time apart for yourself after the birth, which is so important for you and your baby.

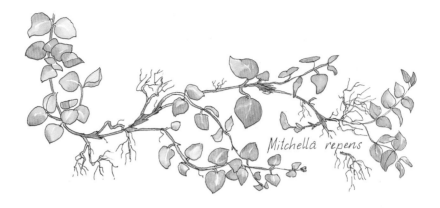

Mitchella repens

RELAXATION
About Relaxation

Deep relaxation

(yoga nidra)

The practice of deep relaxation is especially valuable during pregnancy and after birth. It is a good way to relax your body, calm your mind and replenish lost energies. When you give yourself some quiet time to relax during pregnancy you are recognising the need to take time out, and honouring yourself in preparation for childbirth and becoming a mother.

What is deep relaxation?

In yogic teachings, deep relaxation is called *yoga nidra* which means 'dynamic sleep'. During *yoga nidra*, the physical body experiences complete relaxation and stillness as if it were sleeping but the mind remains alert and awake. The level of awareness of the mind is far deeper than in the normal resting state. Deeper, more expansive and less limited realms of the self are revealed. This deep state of mind lies somewhere between being awake and being asleep, somewhere between your concious and your unconscious mind and far beyond your normal range of awareness.

During deep relaxation you will gradually become more detached from the outside environment and the usual chatter of your mind, as your senses are withdrawn. You come to rest in a remarkable place inside yourself where true peace and quiet can be found. Once this space has been accessed, you will experience the absolute joy of stillness in your body and clearness of thought, with a focused awareness that is entirely absorbed in the present moment. It is here, in this space deep within your own being, that your most peaceful feelings will be discovered and explored.

Yoga Nidra is the doorway to Samadi.

(Swami Satyananda 1978)

Samadi is a state where there is

158

The complete book of
yoga and meditation
for pregnancy

only the experience of joy, pure consciousness and truth, and where the practitioner is at one with the object of his or her meditation. B. K. S. Iyengar (1966) speaks of *samadi* in the introduction to his book *Light on Yoga*. He said, 'There is a peace that surpasseth all understanding. . . the state can only be expressed by profound silence. . . The Yogi has departed from the material world and is merged in the Eternal.' (p. 52) I feel this profound statement more fully explains the feeling of this state and its true essence. Only by spending time in deep relaxation and meditation can we begin to glimpse what the great teachers are really describing.

The value of deep relaxation

It is widely accepted that the value of deep relaxation goes beyond relieving fatigue and tiredness. When deep relaxation is practised regularly, balance and harmony are replenished and maintained through all levels of the person giving your soul, mind and body time to heal more completely.

These days it seems we have become conditioned to keep on going until we are forced to stop either by the appearance of physical symptoms or signs of emotional stress. It is not uncommon for people to feel guilty if they take time out to relax or sleep during the day, even when they are totally exhausted and desperately in need of a break. Difficult times are encountered in every person's life and some are definitely more extreme than others but the more skilled you become at relieving stress, staying calm and making time available for regular relaxation the more likely you are to survive the ordeals of life with a degree of grace and with your health intact.

It is far better to become familiar with relaxation techniques and to take the time out to re-energise yourself regularly than to wait until exhaustion, illness or stress take hold. Often, without deep relaxation, medicines take longer to be effective or they simply mask the true cause of the illness. I feel that all other therapies are enriched when time is given to being quiet and still. Taking time out from life's physical demands or from emotional overload is simply an act of nurturing yourself.

Making relaxation a habit in your life is like having an in-built insurance scheme because the more time you invest in maintaining a balanced life, the greater the rewards will be in the long term.

Deep relaxation is especially beneficial during pregnancy and after birth but also when you are tired, if you have high blood pressure, if you suffer regular headaches or are under stress. Even if you are already very relaxed and the type of person who never gets ruffled or unhinged, you will still benefit from deep relaxation as it is a complete therapy in itself.

Many of us seek to know peace and calmness and are constantly searching outside ourselves to fulfill those desires and to satisfy our restless needs. However, through the practice of deep relaxation, we come to realise we need only look outside ourselves for guidance and to learn the skills, as it is within ourselves that true clarity and quietness dwell.

The postures

There are five relaxation postures suitable for pregnancy and all of them are simple to do and gentle on your body. The position of your body has a big influence on your ability to relax completely, so it is important to select a posture that is comfortable for you.

The first two postures can be used during your yoga practices, at night in bed or when you need to rest during the day. They are designed to allow your muscles to release tension so that your body begins to feel as if it is sinking into the floor or floating lightly and weightlessly.

The remaining three postures induce calmness in your mind and are also good for removing discomfort in your shoulder and back muscles. Even though these three postures are designed for relaxation rather than for their physical benefits, they also gently stretch your whole spinal column and release unwanted tension in those parts of the body.

It will be a matter of trying each of these positions for yourself, to establish the most comfortable one to use at different stages of your pregnancy. However, your preferred posture could change throughout your pregnancy depending on how you are feeling and how the baby is lying in the womb.

General instructions
- When you practise deep relaxation always lie on a soft but firm surface that is away from draughts and other disturbances.
- Make sure you will be completely comfortable for the intended relaxation time. Some people like to place a low pillow or cushion under their head for extra comfort.
- If the weather is cool, cover yourself with a blanket and wear socks as your body temperature will naturally drop when you relax. If possible, remain quite still for the whole relaxation.
- There are many tapes available for the purpose of relaxation. Having one of your own enables you to

practise in the comfort and privacy of your home.
- The time given to relaxation can be anywhere from a few minutes to around half an hour.

1. The Corpse
(shavasana)

The Corpse posture is the classic yoga posture for relaxation and it is suitable for the early months of pregnancy. Preferably, it is done with your legs slightly bent but it can also be done with your legs straight. If you have back problems small cushions or folded blankets can be placed in the curve of your back and behind your knees to ease discomfort.

Doctors usually recommend this posture be discontinued as the pregnancy progresses because lying on your back puts pressure on the major veins leading to the fetus, often resulting in nausea and discomfort. Most women find that by around 15 weeks of pregnancy the Flapping Fish posture is more comfortable for both relaxing and sleeping. This posture is an ideal way to feel the relaxation response throughout your whole body.

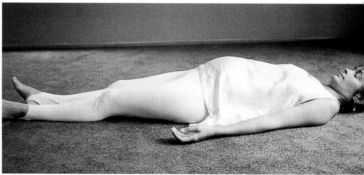

1. Lie on a comfortable surface with your head and back supported. Cover your body with a light rug or blanket.

2. Relax your face and lightly close your eyes. Let your teeth rest a little apart and relax your jaw. Allow

160

The complete book of
yoga and meditation
for pregnancy

your lips to rest in a soft smile and be sure that your forehead is free from frowning.

3. Rest your arms a little away from your body, your palms turned upwards and your thumbs and index fingers joined in *chin mudra*.

4. Rest your legs slightly apart and allow your feet to fall freely to the sides.

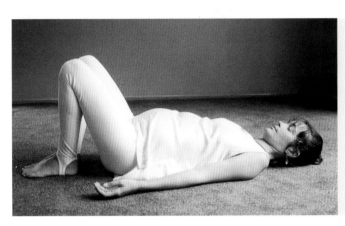

5. Straighten your spine so that your shoulders and hips are in line. Point your chin slightly into the centre of your chest to prevent pressure on your neck.

6. Breathe quietly and gently and feel the peace and calmness on all levels. Feel the deep relaxation in your body and mind.

2. The Flapping Fish
(matsya kridasana)

The Flapping Fish is a very comfortable posture to use when the Corpse posture becomes uncomfortable, especially later in your pregnancy. Many pregnant women sleep in this position and it is especially useful if your back is sore.

For comfort, place a pillow under your bent knee and under your abdomen to ease pressure on your back. Full body-length pillows are available from some department stores and bedding specialist and these are ideal to

use during relaxation. This relaxation posture is particularly beneficial if you have sciatica problems because the nerves to your legs are relaxed. The pelvic area is lightly stretched which gently stimulates your digestive system, and time spent in this posture sometimes relieves mild constipation. Once in this posture it is extremely relaxing and is suitable for use throughout pregnancy.

1. Lie on your right side with your head resting on a pillow or on your arm.

2. Leave your right leg straight but bend your left leg so that it rests comfortably on the floor or on a pillow.

3. Your left arm can rest on the floor, or you might like to place your

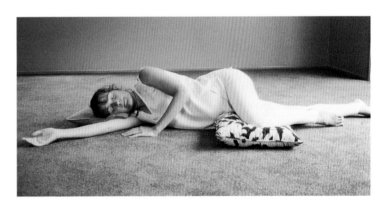

hand on your abdomen to feel the movements of your baby in your womb. Adjust your position and pillows to suit your own needs.

4. Lying on your right side will stimulate the more passive left side of your brain. This means that relaxation is more quickly induced because your mind is less bothered by unwanted thoughts. This is useful to remember for labour as a reliable and easy way to become more relaxed and centred. This posture can also be used lying on the left side of your body.

3. The Pose of the Child
(sishuasana)

This posture was named the Pose of the Child because it resembles the fetal position and because it is not uncommon to see small children sleeping this way, totally relaxed and at peace. A short time spent in this posture will bring quietness to your mind, a slowing down of thoughts, quieter breathing and a relaxed body. It is a wonderful posture to do if your mind is overloaded with unwanted thoughts or if it seems impossible to rest. With your head placed either on the floor or on your folded hands, there is an increased blood flow to your head gently stimulating the relaxation centres of your brain.

Some people relax more in the Pose of the Child than the two previous postures because it creates a feeling of safety and nurturing. You will notice your breathing slowing down the longer you hold the posture. If you are in an all-fours position during labour, relaxing into the Pose of the Child or a similar posture between contractions is very restful and also beneficial to the mood of your labour.

This posture is suitable for the first two or three months of pregnancy. As your pregnancy progresses, your knees can be moved further apart to accommodate the increasing size of your abdomen. In this posture you will notice a deep stretch to your inner thigh area. When your knees are wider than your feet it becomes the Pose of the Hare.

This posture is especially useful at times of anxiety and mental confusion. It is also beneficial for headaches which are often caused by stress and tension. It is important to note there are no contraindications for people with high blood pressure, even though your head is down and below your heart. The Pose of the Child has proven to be a favourite posture for many people.

1. Begin by sitting in the Thunderbolt posture (detailed in the chapter, 'Warming up'). Bring your body forward and rest your forehead on the floor. Keep your eyes lightly closed.

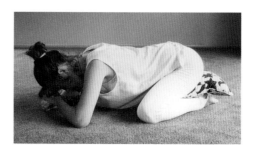

2. Rest your arms alongside your body so that your hands are near your feet. Alternatively, rest your head on your folded hands. If you have knee or ankle problems, one or two small cushions can be placed between the back of your thighs and your calf muscles, and under your feet. This is particularly important if you have varicose veins.

3. Depending on your size and stage of pregnancy, your knees can either be kept together or spread apart. When your knees are wider apart, you may also like to place a small cushion under your abdomen to prevent a curve forming in the middle of your back.

4. The final posture can be held for as long as desired, breathing quietly and relaxing deeply into the posture.

4. The Pose of the Hare

The Pose of the Hare is very similar to the previous posture. From mid-pregnancy on, however, it will accommodate your growing shape better than the Pose of the Child.

1. The only difference between the two postures is that for the Hare your knees are opened as wide as you

162

The complete book of
yoga and meditation
for pregnancy

personally find comfortable, and your arms are stretched out beyond your head. Many women notice a lovely stretch throughout the length of the back and an 'opening' across the lower back and pelvic areas when resting in the Pose of the Hare.

2. It is recommended to use this

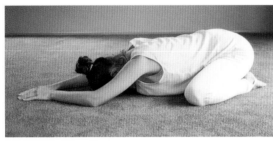

posture to rest between contractions during labour. It is also an ideal posture for lower back massage during labour. As your pelvis is tilted slightly upwards, your baby will rest further up into your birth canal and this often proves to be of great value in situations where the contractions need to be slowed down or if cervical swelling is causing problems.

5. The Sleeping Tortoise
(supta kurmasana)

The Sleeping Tortoise is similar to the Pose of the Child as it is very easy to do and is most suitable for pregnancy. The small number of people who are not relaxed in the Child or the Hare postures will usually find this more to their liking. However, for those women who are shorter in the body or who are carrying their baby higher under the ribs, the Sleeping Tortoise could feel a bit cramped later in pregnancy. It will be a matter of trying each of these positions for yourself, to establish the most comfortable position to use at different stages of your pregnancy.

In a similar way to the Child, this posture will deeply relax your whole

body and mind making this a very effective posture to relieve all types of mental and emotional stress. The pelvic area, hips and inner thighs are toned and your abdominal area is gently massaged. The longer the posture is held the more your back muscles relax and your inner thigh area opens

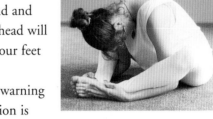

allowing your body to unfold and move into the forward bend and the closer your head will come towards your feet and the floor.

My only warning about this position is that if you stay in it too long you might go to sleep!

1. Sit with the soles of your feet together, a little further away from your body than in the Butterfly posture. Relax your knees and allow them to fall towards the floor. There is no need to force your knees close to the floor in this posture. It is more important that your body is relaxed.

2. Place your hands on top of your feet, or pass them through your legs to rest beside your feet. Ease your body towards your feet into a gentle forward bend.

3. Relax your head and neck and keep your arms free and loose from your shoulders. Bend your elbows slightly.

4. Close your eyes and breathe quietly while you hold the posture. Be aware that your back, shoulders, arms and hands are relaxed at all times as we often tense the body without even realising it. As a general guide, this posture is held for nine breaths but if you're really enjoying yourself, stay there as long as you remain relaxed and comfortable. Counting your breaths is excellent for improving your concentration and it also prevents your mind from wandering.

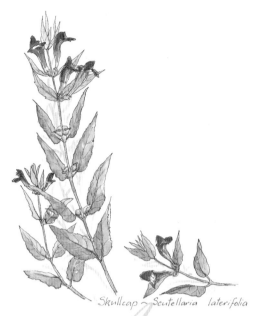

Skullcap ~ Scutellaria laterifolia

ANTENATAL PROGRAMS
Six Half-hour Programs

Clients and students often ask me for a specific, individualised program that can be done between classes. With so many exercises and practices to choose from, it can become confusing deciding which ones to do, especially if you are new to yoga. For many people, a structured, well-balanced program is an ideal way to become familiar with the various practices and techniques, and ultimately to achieve more enjoyment from yoga. Once you have the basic format in mind, and recognise how to put it all together, you can then create your own programs to suit your own requirements.

Follow all the guidelines and precautions recommended and, if necessary, adjust what I have proposed to suit your needs at the time. Always remember to be adaptable and flexible with yourself. Sometimes you might feel fatigued and would prefer to spend

more time meditating or in deep relaxation, rather than concentrating on the postures. That is completely acceptable.

These half-hour programs, consist of gentle exercises which you will find fully detailed in the relevant chapters of the book. Even if you are attending regular classes, it will be a lot easier to continue practising at home with the aid of these separate programs. They are well balanced and easy to follow 'mini' yoga routines, and are designed for you to use whenever you have the time or feel inclined to do them.

Getting started

Always begin with a short relaxation, followed by some slow, deep yoga breathing. If you are in the first trimester, lie on your back with your knees bent, or if you are further along in your pregnancy lay on your side for more comfort. Follow the rhythm of

164

The complete book of
yoga and meditation
for pregnancy

your natural breath flowing evenly and gently in and out of your body. Spend between five and ten minutes relaxing, breathing, and getting in touch with your pregnancy and with your baby.

When you are ready, breathe slowly and deeply four or five times. Notice how you are feeling and use your breathing to release any tension or uneasy emotions, replacing them with a more positive atmosphere that is encouraging to health and wellbeing. Think about how you would prefer to be feeling, and draw in these calming, balanced energies. When you do this before your yoga practice, you will be better prepared with a clearer mind and a more centred attitude.

When you are relaxed and centred, proceed with the programs. I suggest also including the Pelvic Floor exercises daily, remembering they can be done anywhere and at any time of the day.

Feel free to change the format of these programs and create your own from the many exercises and postures in the book. Most importantly, enjoy your yoga and your pregnancy.

Program 1

1. Warming Up: Hand and Finger exercises, Shoulder exercises, Pelvic Rocking.
2. Spinal Twists: The Easy Spinal Twist.
3. Balancing: The Tree.
4. Standing: The Heavenly Stretch, the Triangle Side Bend, the Warrior, the Hero.
5. Relaxing: The Pose of the Child, or the Pose of the Hare.
6. Pranayama: Alternate Nostril Breathing, the Cooling Breath.
7. Relaxing: Deep relaxation by yourself, or play a 10 minute relaxation tape if you have access to one.

Program 2

1. Warming Up: Head and Neck exercises, Shoulder exercises, Hamstring stretches.
2. Standing: Arm stretching, Chest Expansion with Deep Breathing.
3. Squatting: The Deep Standing Squat, the Moving Squat. Any other squatting exercises and *asanas*.
4. Warming Up: The Cat, Pelvic Rocking (on your knees), the Tiger.
5. Relaxation: The Pose of the Hare.
6. Pranayama: Alternate Nostril Breathing, *ujjayi pranayama*.
7. Mediation or deep relaxation.

Program 3

1. Warming Up: Ankle exercises, Hip Rotations, the Half Butterfly, the Butterfly.
2. Floor Postures and Exercise: The Seated Triangle (Stretching over each leg), the Pelvic Tilt.
3. Spinal Twist: Any seated or lying down spinal twist of your choice.
4. Pranayama: Any breathing exercises of your choice.
5. Deep relaxation.

Program 4

1. Warming Up: Any of the warming up exercises.
2. Balancing: the Tree, the Eagle, the Crane, the Dancer. Rest between these postures and before continuing on.
3. Standing: The Wide-A Leg Stretch, the Mountain.
4. Relaxation: The Pose of the Hare.
5. Pranayama: Alternate Nostril Breathing, the Humming Breath
6. Meditation with *ujjayi pranayama*.
7. Relaxation: Deep relaxation.

Program 5

1. Warming Up: Any exercises of your choice.
2. Leg & Abdomen Exercises: Single Leg Lifts, the Infinite Pose (both sides), Single Leg Lifts lying on your back, Gentle Abdominal exercises.
3. Floor Postures & Exercises: The Pelvic Tilt.
4. Spinal Twists: Any seated or lying down spinal twist of your choice.
5. Pranayama: The Humming Breath, the Cooling Breath, *ujjayi pranayama*.
6. Deep relaxation and meditation.

Program 6

1. Squatting: Wall Stretches (the Butterfly, the Wide Leg Stretch).
2. Spinal Twists: Any seated or lying down spinal twist of your choice.
3. Warming Up: The Cat, the Tiger, Pelvic Rocking (on your knees).
4. Relaxation: The Pose of the Hare.
5. Pranayama: Three breathing exercises of your choice.
6. Deep relaxation or meditation.

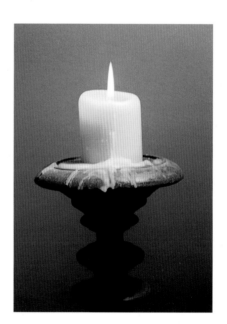

166

The complete book of
yoga and meditation
for pregnancy

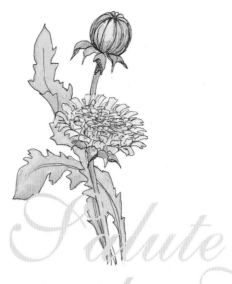

Salute to the Sun for Pregnancy
(surya namaskara)

Over the years of working with pregnant women, I have seen many women continue with this exercises, in complete comfort and ease, right up to their due date. When the Salute to the Sun is practised quietly and sensibly, with careful attention to the precautions and modifications, it is of great benefit to your wellbeing and level of fitness.

Originally, I had not intended to include the Salute to the Sun as part of the antenatal exercises program because of my concerns that some women might overextend themselves and not take enough notice of the precautions and modifications. It seems to be part of human nature to try that little bit harder – even during pregnancy – and although this is a safe and rather passive exercise to do, if the modifications are not followed carefully and the practice is 'overdone' during pregnancy, the result could be exhaustion or

unnecessary straining. This situation is definitely not appropriate during pregnancy and I am trusting it will not be the case when it is included in your antenatal yoga program.

Generally, I find most pregnant women are rather reluctant to give up this practice. Other than the precautions and modifications recommended here, the details and benefits are similar to the standard procedure outlined later in this book. For pregnancy, however, it is done very slowly and quietly.

Precautions

1. Only practise *surya namaskara* if you are enjoying it and feel it is suitable for you personally. At no time should there be any nausea, straining, shortness of breath, dizziness or any other uncomfortable feelings during or after practising.

2. The practice is to be done slowly and quietly, moving from one

posture to the next very gently, especially from the head down positions to the standing positions. It is very important to remember to always come up slowly. If you have high or low blood pressure either seek skilled professional advice or discontinue the exercise completely.

3. Discontinue with the exercise when your size is making you uncomfortable or even if something like the hot summer weather is causing you to feel unwell. If there has been an alteration in your health and general wellbeing you should also avoid this exercise. If there comes a time when this exercise is more of a struggle than a pleasure, it would be better to discontinue it, as obviously it is no longer of benefit to you.

Modifications

- In position 1, your feet should be a little apart rather than together.
- In position 2, do not lean back. Reach your arms up above your head, so that your body is held straight.
- In position 3, some people like to keep their knees slightly bent in the forward bend which is repeated again in position 9. This will relieve pressure on your lower back and hamstrings.
- From position 5, come down onto your knees into the 'all-fours' position. Remember to keep your back straight or parallel with the floor and not swayed. If you like, the Cat stretch can be practised from this position. From here, continue on to position 8 of the standard practice.
- Always practise Salute to the Sun in a quiet and gentle manner, holding each position for two or three breaths to prevent you rushing

through the exercise and to gain the most benefits from the individual postures.

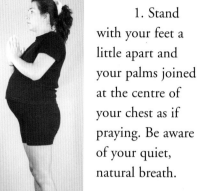

Procedure

1. Stand with your feet a little apart and your palms joined at the centre of your chest as if praying. Be aware of your quiet, natural breath.

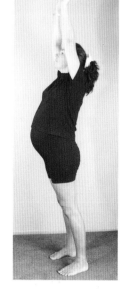

2. Breathe in as you lift your arms above your head, stretching throughout your spine. Keep your shoulders down and relaxed. Remember not to lean back.

3. Breathe out as you slowly bring your body forward so that the top of your head is facing the floor and your upper body falls relaxed from your hips and shoulders. Hold your legs straight. Remain in this position while you breathe gently.

4. When you are ready – or after two or three breaths – take your right leg back, placing your right knee and toes on the floor. Lean forward over

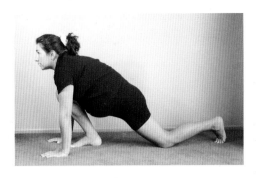

your left knee and rest your hands on either side of your left foot. Hold this posture while you relax and breathe quietly. If the arm position is uncomfortable, place both hands inside your left foot instead of on either side of your foot.

5. Breathe out as you move your left foot back to meet your right foot.

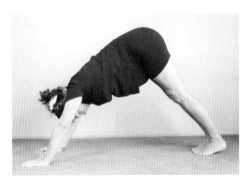

Lift your hips into the Mountain posture. Relax your neck and let your head drop down between your shoulders. Press your heels towards the floor and extend back from your hips. Hold the posture while you breathe quietly. This is more strenuous than the other positions so take care not to strain or hold it for too long. Take particular care in the head down positions if your

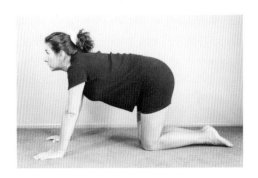

blood pressure is abnormal.

6. Ease down onto your knees into an all-fours position, keeping your back straight. Breathe in as you look ahead. Breathe out as you arch your back, tucking your tail bone under and bringing your chin into your chest to

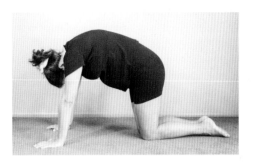

complete the Cat posture.

7. Return to the Mountain posture as you exhale. Breathe gently while you hold the position.

8. Breathe in as you move your left leg forward, repeating position 4.

9. Breathe out as you bring both feet together and straighten your legs. Let your head hang down as for position 3, and your knees can be bent slightly if that is more comfortable.

10. Breathe in as you slowly stand up. Gradually stretch your arms up above your head as in position 2.

11. Breathe out and return to position 1, with your palms together at the centre of your chest.

This completes half of one round of Salute to the Sun. One round is where the exercise is repeated as above, only in positions 4 and 8 the opposite leg is extended back.

Repeat this exercise if you are not out of breath or tired. When you have finished the exercise, rest on the floor – preferably with your knees bent – for a short relaxation until your breathing and your heart rate have returned to normal.

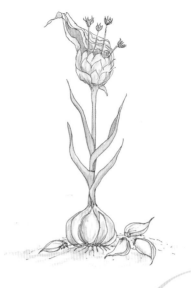

BIRTH
My Story

The idea for this book was conceived when I was pregnant with my first son Ezra. I had been practising yoga for many years and continuing on with it during pregnancy seemed the logical thing to do. At that time I was fortunate enough to be under the guidance of an excellent teacher, Swami Shantimurti. I knew the time to conceive was drawing near so I spoke to him about a specific yoga program that would prepare my body for conception and the changes that would occur during pregnancy. I wanted to be as healthy and strong as I could be before conception, not only through a healthy diet and lifestyle but also with the assistance of yoga.

I was one of those lucky people who had decided to conceive in three months time and I did just that. At that time I was also completing my naturopathic studies at a college in Auckland. To qualify, I was required to do a thesis. I remember knowing that I had to do mine on yoga and pregnancy and I was thrilled when Angela, the lecturer in charge of thesis topics, accepted my choice.

And so began my long journey with this book which I feel has symbolically gone through its own pregnancy, time *in utero*, and birth. To complete more studies in Australia I provided an enlarged and more detailed update of the original thesis, which became the background for this book. In many ways the book has had its own growth *in utero* as it slowly took form over time, growing and developing, maturing and becoming whole, until its 'birth' when it was finally completed.

My own experience with yoga began in Melbourne where I attended classes for some years. Later on, I had the opportunity to delve deeper while travelling in India – particularly in the extraordinary city of Bombay – and

Ezra

later while living in London. After returning to Australia for a brief time, I moved to New Zealand and unexpectedly found myself teaching a large group in a provincial town, which continued for a couple of years before moving to Auckland where I met my most influential teacher, Shantimurti.

My initiation into teaching yoga for pregnancy seemed to come about as something I was meant to do rather than something I had the time to actually consider. After a happy and healthy pregnancy and a fairly straightforward birth with Ezra, my doctor suggested – while I was still in the delivery room – that I start classes for pregnant women as soon as I was ready. It was not really something I was thinking about 15 minutes after giving birth! However, his suggestion turned, within a few months, into a small class of women all referred by him. That was some 15 years ago.

My second son, Reuben, was to have quite a different experience from

his brother both *in utero* and for his birth. We were living aboard our yacht when I conceived and we were sailing the Pacific during the last five months of his pregnancy. Due to engine problems we were forced to stop for repairs at the island of Espiritu Santo in northern Vanuatu. I was about 30 weeks.

On visiting the rather basic and unsophisticated local hospital there – which is as polite as I can be – I was told by the local doctor that he would not interfere with the birth as this was the domain of the midwives and that there were no analgesics handed out for normal deliveries. He also told me no real fuss was made about labour and birth in Vanuatu because women had babies all the time and they just got on with it as well as they could! Although I realise that giving birth and having babies is a very natural part of life and something that happens all the time, it's still a bit of a shock when it's as simplified as that.

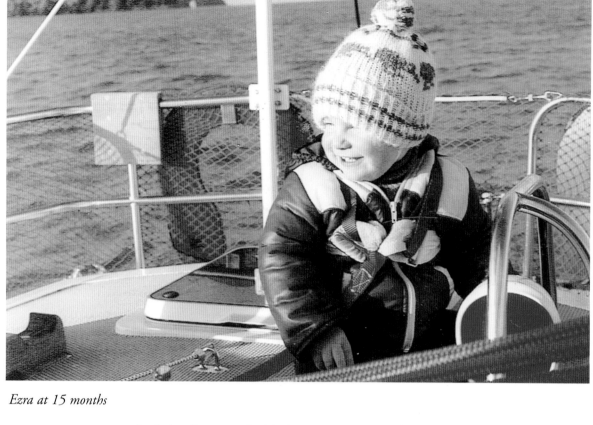

Ezra at 15 months

So, being forewarned with the reality of the situation, I armed myself with all the skills I knew, practising my yoga postures and especially the breathing exercises intensely for the remaining 10 weeks of my pregnancy.

I also knew that it was considered taboo for men to be present at the birth and without that support from my husband, Jeff, I had to find all the strength I needed from within myself. With this to consider I relied heavily on meditation and visualisation techniques, as well as plain positive thinking, all of which I feel played a big part in what turned out to be a very straightforward delivery. Maybe I was lucky, but I know I would not have handled such unusual circumstances – or been so relaxed – if I had not physically, and most importantly, mentally and emotionally, prepared myself beforehand.

I have warm and pleasant memories of the day Reuben was born.

I was feeling very much in control of what was happening. I felt so calm as I progressed through the contractions, completely focused on my breathing and going with the whole process. I was definitely helped out by nature on that cool September evening. For most of the first stage I was on the beach where the yacht was moored then, later that evening, I moved through the more intense contractions on the hill outside the hospital which overlooked the sea. All the while, I was being cooled by a light breeze that swayed the coconut palms.

To some people this might seem a rather bizarre and unconventional way to be in labour but it was very pleasing to my inner being and soothing to my soul. I was able to become absorbed in the natural birthing processes and connect with my inner feminine wisdom, in a beautiful natural setting.

At the time, I think I would have

The complete book of
yoga and meditation
for pregnancy

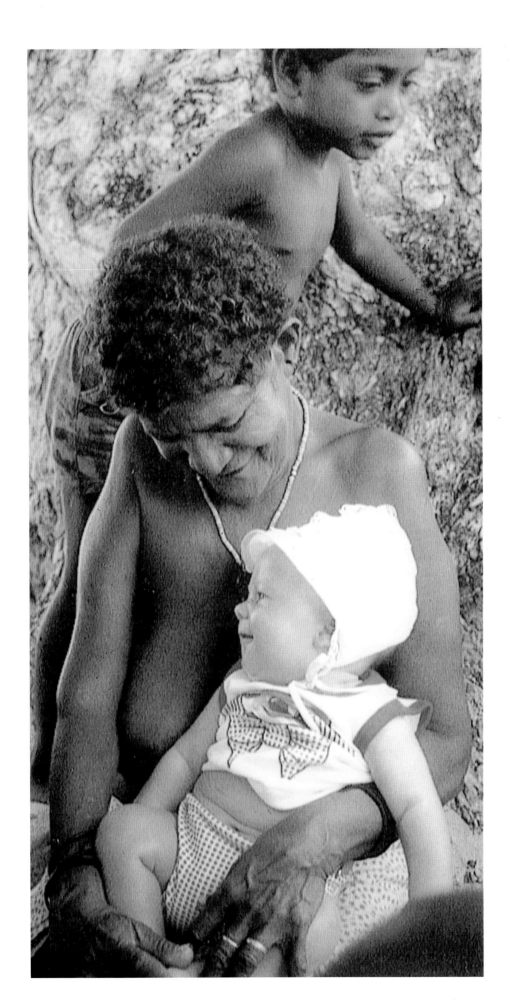

*Reuben with a
Solomon Islander*

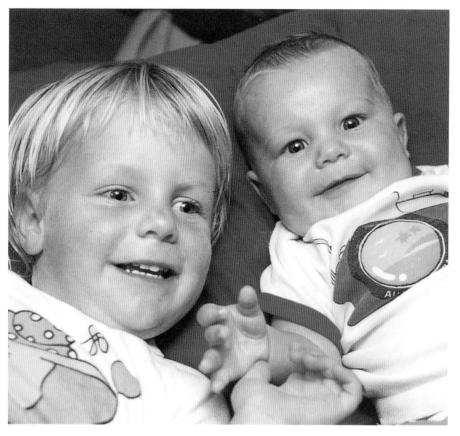

Ezra and Reuben

welcome aboard. Reuben lived the first 10 months of his life on the water before we moved back onto land and it was not long after that I began teaching again.

I often wonder at how fortunate I am to be in the remarkable position of teaching yoga as a profession. It is especially an honour to teach women at such a unique and precious time in their lives. Not only do I love this work and see it more as a blessing than a job, but it has also given me the opportunity to meet and make close friends with many beautiful and inspiring women, who have taught me more than I feel I have taught them. Of course, there is the additional joy of finally meeting their newborns, often only days after being born. It is always a very emotional experience for me after observing them move and grow in their mother's abdomen for so long.

These are my stories, in brief. Without doubt every mother has their own unique birth story, all very different and each an event in itself. For this reason I have included a special chapter dedicated to personal birth journeys, in which 11 very different women have shared their special moments and thoughts about how yoga played a significant role during pregnancy and in preparation for labour and birth, as well as how valuable the different techniques proved to be after the birth.

been quite happy to have stayed where I was because it really was peaceful but the midwife was more practical than me and insisted on me coming inside. Even though it was not a completely ideal situation – in that I had to go it alone without the support of Jeff – I knew I was safe and I am glad for the experience. I am especially glad for the knowledge that yoga played such a big role in helping me manage as well as I did.

There were definitely no luxuries offered at that small hospital, not even a cup of tea or a warm shower after the delivery. So, we came back to the boat early the next day for a peaceful time together with our new family member on the still waters of Pelacula Bay. Although we had no family or friends there to visit us and welcome Reuben to the world, we did receive radio calls from other boats in the Pacific area, wishing us all well and Reuben

The complete book of
yoga and meditation
for pregnancy

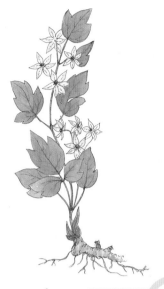

Birth Journeys

For me, pregnancy was an initiatory experience that changed my body, shifted my consciousness, taught me surrender, and was the beginning of the dawning awareness of the physical, psychological, and spiritual demands and gifts that would come through being a mother.

(Bolen 1994, p. 53)

It is my great pleasure to include these very personal stories from women who have practiced yoga during their pernancies. As you will see from reading the stories, some women were very involved in yoga for the entire pregnancy, while others only discovered it during the last few months. Yet, all felt it played an important role in many different ways. It is a privilege to make their special journeys available to share with others and I hope they will prove to be valuable and insightful reading while you prepare for the birth of your baby.

When you are pregnant, it is very helpful to listen to other women speak about their birth experiences, especially how other women coped and handled the different stages of labour. It can help to build confidence and courage for your own special journey. Obviously, there will be some labour stories that won't be as easy to listen to as others, being a fact of life that some women have an easier time giving birth than others. However, not all birth experiences are horrific. In fact, for some women, giving birth is one of 'the' remarkable events in their life. For this reason, I encourage women to listen to all stories, including the inevitable horror stories which people seem so eager to tell, but also to seek out women who had a more positive and fulfilling time giving birth, and to draw strength from their encouraging stories. Finding the balance between all the possibilities of pregnancy, labour and childbirth, and being in touch with the realities of life, will make you more aware of what could happen and prepare you for your own individual circumstance.

1. Debbie's story: The birth of Callan

As this was my first child, I wanted to prepare myself as best as one can, and I felt yoga would be the most ideal way to cater to the mental and physical demands of pregnancy and childbirth.

I joined Theresa's yoga group at about 18 weeks into my pregnancy. The classes were designed for pregnancy, so the postures, meditation and relaxation techniques were ideally suited and specific to the needs of an advancing pregnancy. Also, you were able to work at your own level and pace which I feel is important.

The benefits were almost immediate, particularly if you were disciplined and practised at home on a daily basis. The interaction with other pregnant ladies was great and also quite social. My intention was to continue the classes until I was due, but mother nature was to chart her own course as I developed Pregnancy Induced Hypertension at 26 weeks.

At 32 weeks I was hospitalised, and the challenge I was faced with was to try and extend my pregnancy for as long as possible. It was at this point that yoga became particularly important for me, as I was surrounded by women having their babies and then going home. Quite the opposite for me however, as I was trying very hard not to have my baby and at the same time pass my time in hospital effectively and positively. So yoga became a very big part of my daily routine in hospital, and as it turned out enabled me

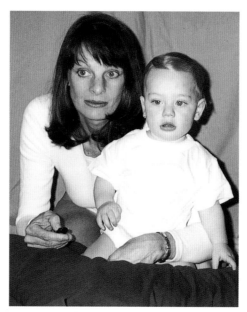

to remain calm mentally, which in turn kept my blood pressure levels sufficiently low to gain valuable weeks for my baby to continue to grow and develop, until I was induced at 36 weeks.

During the initial stages of labour, I walked a lot and then retired to the spa in the birthing suite and seriously concentrated on the breathing techniques I had learnt at the yoga classes. I choose to spend a lot of this time alone, which allowed my mind to be incredibly focused and clear and afforded me a degree of control physically, to work with the contractions as my labour progressed to the transitional stage. At this point, I left the spa and tried various positions on the floor, maintaining my breathing the whole time. From transition to the actual birth, everything proceeded very quickly and my husband and girlfriend joined me to witness the wondrous moment our baby boy arrived, healthy and beautiful. My labour was drug free which amazed me, as I am certainly no martyr and had decided, in advance, to take pain relief if and when I needed it.

A few days after the birth my midwife asked me if I would speak to her current antenatal class before I went home. I inquired why, and she told me that I had gone into a trance-like state as soon as I got into the spa, concentrating on deep breathing, and remaining that way the entire time. She felt it was my knowledge of yoga that rewarded me with a very easy labour, as labour goes, and wanted me to share this with her class,

176

The complete book of
yoga and meditation
for pregnancy

which I did happily. Upon reflection, I now realise what an 'outer body experience' my labour had been, even though I was not aware of this at the time.

To be honest I thought my yoga had served its purpose during pregnancy and labour, so I moved on to the busy days ahead caring for our son, Callan. No one can really prepare you for labour, you must experience it. The same applies to the first weeks at home, when the days roll into nights of very little sleep and you seem to merely exist for your baby, constantly wondering if what you are doing is correct, while at the same time becoming familiar with your baby. It is during these early weeks you are really tested mentally and physically. Once again yoga came to my rescue and I was able to draw on my ability through meditation to remain calm mentally, and the relaxation techniques boosted me physically and emotionally.

Overall, I am convinced yoga was my saviour at times when I needed it most and still is on a daily basis, proving to me the benefits of yoga don't cease with labour. Applied daily or as often as time allows, yoga in all its forms continues to feed the mind, body and soul, at a time when our lives become so busy and stressful. In turn this flows on to contribute to a contented baby, so mother and father can both be more relaxed to enjoy the new role of parenting. I feel everyone should have access to the benefits of yoga if they so desire, especially during pregnancy.

2. Eva's Birth Experience

Ella's journey into the world stirred in me the deepest and most unexpected of emotions. I firmly believed in having an active birth and had prepared myself from the beginning of my pregnancy by reading whatever books I could find on active birth experiences. I was quite sure of what I wanted – no drugs, for example, and the freedom to move about and take up what ever position I wanted. As it turned out, things did not happen as expected and, in the end, medical intervention was, for me, not only necessary but even welcome.

Leaning forward into the back of a

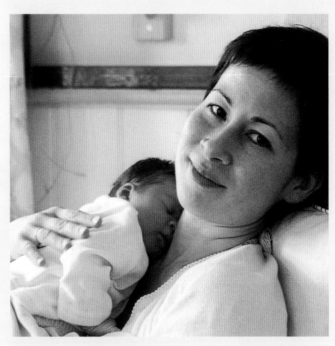

chair throughout my entire labor, I refused to move. Yet despite the physical intensity of labour, I felt remarkably calm and at peace with myself – a feeling I attribute largely to yoga and meditation practices which had become an essential part of my daily routine months before the birth. Practising yoga and meditation regularly helped me enormously in gathering my focus and centering my energy when I required it most. I imagined myself riding the crest of a wave with each contraction, knowing it would eventually subside. With the help of my partner and close girlfriend who offered continued encouragement, bringing me back to my point of focus when I appeared to be drifting, I was thus able to manage my contractions. At the most intense point of my labour, however, a very specific visualisation technique I had learnt in yoga unexpectedly came to me. I imagined myself enclosed in a pyramid, where nothing could harm me and, as my contractions increased, I found myself thinking of a spiral lifting me out of my physical body, through the top of the pyramid. It was a very powerful experience, especially considering I did not particularly take to this practice during the actual yoga classes.

I look back at my birth experience as a joyous one. While the labour itself was difficult it shall always remain captured in my memory in the most emotionally positive way.

3. Veronica's baby, Amber Mae.

When I found out I was pregnant with my fourth child, I was in shock. Not only was I a busy career mum with three active children, I was also newly separated from my husband. I had promised myself that I would never go through labour again, as my other three experiences had

been long and tedious, the last one being over 30 hours long and extremely painful. I couldn't believe that I had to face it all again . . . and this time on my own.

After the panic had subsided I decided to confront the problem. I began by researching all aspects of childbirth so as to ease the agony that I felt I was sure to endure. It was my favourite aunt who suggested yoga, and desperate as I was I decided to give it a go, anything could help. I was fortunate to have first called Theresa, who ran classes for pregnancy.

From the first class I knew I had found the answer, as yoga was everything I was looking for. The exercises were perfect for my changing body, they felt really great, and the meditations did wonders for my mind. I was starting to feel fit and well, both physically and mentally. I continued to do the stretches and the meditations at home throughout the week and looked forward to the next class. Most importantly, I felt confident that I would at least survive my approaching ordeal.

And survive I did. The breathing exercises that had been so beneficial during my pregnancy proved fabulous during my labour, keeping me both relaxed and focused, while the deep relaxation was exactly what I needed during pregnancy and especially during labour. The most amazing aspect of the whole ordeal was the fact that my labour was only one and a quarter hours long from start to finish. I barely made it to the delivery suite, when my healthy baby girl Amber Mae arrived into the world. While labour would by no means be my most favourite experience in life, I can clearly say that yoga was of

The complete book of
yoga and meditation
for pregnancy

great benefit to me, making the birth easier, quicker and bearable.

My recovery was also aided by yoga, as I continued on with some gentle stretching exercises and pelvic floor exercises, as well as listening to my relaxation tapes and doing my yoga breathing. I have since been proclaiming the benefits that yoga has had on all aspects of childbirth and I can highly recommend it to any pregnant mum. Actually, I recommend it to any mum, as the techniques that got me through labour, are also an important part of coping with the day to day stresses of being a mother, especially if you're a single mother to four active children and moving along the challenging path of recreating a career.

Yoga has been an amazing experience for my family and me, and I know it will be great for others too.

4. The birth of Ebony-Jayne

My son was born 10 years earlier in a relatively short time, lasting only four hours from the first twinge of labour to less than an hour for the second stage, and all my friends teased me saying I needed to experience a 'real birth'. Even though at that time, I was extremely fit and had been active up until the birth, I found that I needed to use gas as I had not learned to calm and control myself during the pregnancy. When it came to the final minutes of the birth, my mind wandered and focused on the pain, hence the tensing of muscles and the need to be cut to allow the baby free. Even though all births are a wonderful experience, taking the time to learn to relax the mind and body throughout this pregnancy, made the comparison between both births obvious.

The birth of our daughter Ebony-Jayne was a wonderful experience, even though my labour lasted a total of 17 hours, definitely a 'real birth', after being induced due to the rise in my blood

pressure. I went into true labour quite excited after a false labour lasting 10 days, when I had lost the mucus plug and had been mildly labouring ever since with several false starts. I was now pleased my contractions were coming at a regular 7 to 10 minutes apart. My labour was progressing slowly and my friend Sharon gave me homeopathic drops, which helped the intensity of the contractions. After trying several positions for labour, I found lying on my side the most comfortable. After much time and really getting nowhere fast, my waters were broken by my doctor and from then on the

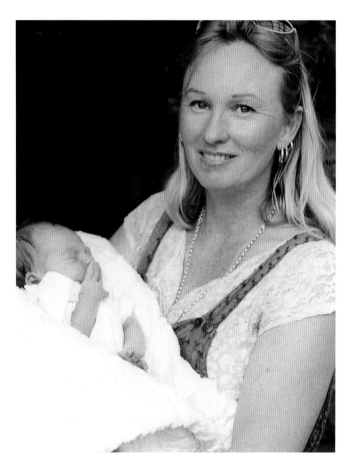

contractions were close together and very intense, as well as the desire to push. I found that the pain was easier to handle on my hands and knees, relaxing into the Pose of the Hare in between contractions to allow the weight and gravity to take the pressure off my back.

At this point there was a change of

shifts and Tina became my midwife, a calm and skilled woman who encouraged me to breathe through the pain of each contraction. I wanted to push, but Tina told me I had at least 10 contractions to go, at which point my strength waned and I felt I couldn't last the distance – really telling myself I can't do this! But I pulled myself together and concentrated on the breathing I had been taught in yoga class, relaxing while breathing in and releasing all pain and discomfort while breathing out. I was able to push the panic I was feeling away, and started to relax as much as possible. Tina was encouraging me all the way, telling me to continue with what I was doing, but if I was to push at that time the baby's head would push against the cervix causing it to swell, which could cause complications if the swelling became too great. I remember Theresa telling me that the Mountain pose was an effective way to relieve that pressure, as it allowed the baby to move slightly away from the cervix, reducing extra pressure and also my desire to push. So at the start of the next contraction in the all fours position, I straightened my legs and breathed and breathed and breathed. The overwhelming desire to push lessened as the baby fell with gravity away from the cervix, and after two more contractions Tina said I could push as I was completely dilated.

So I began to push and after several contractions my husband Brett said, 'I can see the head'. With Sharon on one side whispering encouragement and Dianne on the other massaging my back to relieve the pain – a pain I can only relate to as a chinese burn, Ebony came into the world with no tears, no stitches or drugs. A healthy 7 lb 2 oz baby girl. They handed my beautiful daughter to me and as I focused on her I felt an enormous resurgence of energy, and I cried tears of love, joy, exhaustion and relief as I realised I had a daughter, Ebony-Jayne.

I then put her to my breast to encourage the birth of the placenta. Ebony's cord had now stopped pulsating and Brett cut the umbilical cord while she was in my arms, the joy and trepidation on his face was obvious as he hesitated, fearing he would hurt this tiny perfect baby who had just been born to us. He then held her in his arms and bonded with her. Tina pressed down onto the abdomen and the placenta was delivered in a few minutes, being a wonderful experience both physically and emotionally, a completion and cleansing after the whole birthing process. I recommend all women be allowed to enjoy this part of birth as naturally as possible, without the use of hormones to hurry on the process. Ebony's placenta is now feeding a Candlenut tree that continues to grow in our yard, Ebony's tree.

I recommend yoga to any pregnant woman, for the benefits it gives to the body and the mind.

Author's note: Tina Neff was the midwife attending Trish, for the birth of Ebony and she wrote this report about the experience.

I had the privilege of assisting Trish and Brett in the birth of their beautiful daughter, Ebony-Jayne. Once Trish was established in labour, she worked extremely well with her support person Dianne. During this time, she was encouraged to remain focused on her breathing and spontaneously changed positions to be on all fours. Even though Trish's labour was intense, she was able to remain in control and focus on her deeper rhythmic breathing. This control and focus certainly did a great deal to aid the process of labour.

Trish did so well with her breathing and focusing, that I would encourage anyone and everyone who is contemplating yoga training during their

The complete book of
yoga and meditation
for pregnancy

pregnancies, to certainly follow it through. Both the inner control and positioning greatly assisted Trish and Brett in achieving a wonderful birth experience.

Trish's support person Dianne, also did a lot of back massage which helped in relaxing the back muscles and shifted the focus off the 'pain'. Stimulating the sacral points also helped to dissipate the pain and shift the centre of focus. A pain that is more 'dilute' and not so concentrated, is easier to deal with and get through.

After being privileged enough to assist Trish and Brett in their labour experience and share the wonderful, joyous moments of Ebony's birth, I would thoroughly and wholeheartedly recommend the practice of yoga and the breathing techniques to everyone. I can see that it not only assists in managing labour and birth, but also aides the person's inner strength and wellbeing.

5. Wendy Allen: Sarah Joy Allen's 'Birth Day'

Sarah's conception was a honeymoon surprise. Delighted as I was, I knew nothing of what to expect of pregnancy or babies. So this was the beginning of an enormous and continuing learning experience. I wanted to have as healthy and natural pregnancy and birth as possible, and I focused on my physical and spiritual wellbeing. Yoga and hypnotherapy played a major part in my preparation program along with a healthy life style, with particular attention to diet and exercise.

Sarah's expected date of arrival, 20th of August, came and went. Rob and I saw our doctor after every five day's, and after two and a half weeks of waiting we decided to induce Sarah on the 6th of September. Over those final days of waiting we exhausted all the natural methods of inducement including hypnotherapy, yoga, acupuncture, massage,

lots of exercise, love making and wishful thinking!

On the evening of the 5th, after checking into the hospital, the nurses inserted the progesterone jelly at 10 p.m. and 4 a.m.. My contractions were slow and I found I was able to use various yoga poses during this time, including the Crow Walking and the Butterfly Pose in particular. At 1 p.m. my doctor arrived and as things were progressing very slowly, my waters were broken and the drip was inserted. I thought I was prepared for this but I found myself feeling very uncomfortable, anxious and fearful. Once

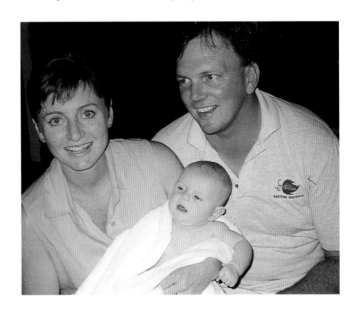

the drip was inserted the show started without me, and the intensity of the pain took me by surprise.

At this time I really wanted a Caesar, but the strength and compassion I found in Joy's voice (the midwife) convinced me I didn't need one or really want one. She gave me the faith and strength I needed in myself and everything changed from that moment on. I realised I had to help myself and that I was going nowhere with my negativity, accepting there was no way out but forward, being strong and positive.

All the techniques I had learnt in the previous months came flooding back to

me, and I became focused on my breathing, finding the ujjayi breathing technique was most valuable. Both the midwives present commented on the ease and depth of the relaxation I was achieving in between contractions. I was able to visualise the opening of my womb and see each contraction as a positive part of the process. Time vanished, I felt removed from those around me and I remember gazing out of the window towards the mountains and feeling very relaxed and dreamy. It was transition, and at this point and I completely surrendered myself, realising nature was taking over, giving the body time to recover and prepare for the next stage of labour.

I soon felt a slight pressure on the anal area as though I needed to move my bowels and after being examined, I was ready to push as I had completely dilated. I got off the bed and into a squatting position leaning over the bed and found I had an incredible urge to push. I was then supported in a squatting position with Rob supporting me from behind. The contractions were at their peak and I felt in control, but not in control – in the sense that nature and instinct had taken over. My mind and body were working as one following their natural course, the inner strength of this process was truly amazing. My throat quickly became sore and hoarse with the effort and I was surprised how physically demanding this was, as I was using all my stamina and strength to stay with it.

The midwife placed a mirror so I could watch the birth, and the sight of Sarah coming into the world is one I will never forget. When she was born she looked surprised laying on her back, arms and legs spread open, obviously wondering what on earth was happening. I couldn't take my eyes off her and Rob cut the cord.

The first touch, the first cuddle, no words can ever describe the awe of this moment. Time seemed to have stopped and I was lost in a state of disbelief gazing at Sarah, before realising I had the daughter I hardly dared to dream of, for wanting too much. She was soon in Rob's arms, a very special time for both of them as they looked at each other for the first time, becoming completely absorbed in one another. We then spent wonderful hours enjoying ourselves snuggling and enjoying the euphoria.

Pregnancy and childbirth have been a truly wonderful experience, one that I feel thankful to have enjoyed. Although it has offered various challenges, none have been as great or demanding as those that are faced now as a new mother, nor as rewarding. Motherhood adds a new dimension to the word 'Love'.

For anyone reading this who is preparing for labour and birth, I could not recommend strongly enough the practice of yoga. It can help you with so many aspects of pregnancy, labour and birth, everything from breathing, relaxation, mental approach, physical suppleness, strength and stamina. It has been, and still is invaluable to me.

6. Lindsay Welch: Morgan's birth

I had been doing yoga throughout my pregnancy and felt really well prepared, relaxed and ready. I had attended my last class when I was more than a week overdue but still did all the postures and enjoyed the class. On the day Morgan was born I woke early with period-like pains, my pelvic floor muscles were tightening and it felt as though a fist was pushing down inside me. At 11.30 I remember thinking to myself that Morgan was going to arrive today!!

The discomfort continued all day and by mid-afternoon the contractions were five minutes apart, although only lasting a short time. I was able to walk *around and was getting very excited at the thought that soon I would see my baby. During Yoga I had often visualised my 'special place' as Fleays nature reserve which is behind our home, and it always made me feel relaxed and close to the beauty of nature. So with it being so close to my home, my husband and I went for a lovely walk to help get things moving.*

Later in the afternoon the contractions were getting much stronger and I was having difficulty coping with backache. I found sitting in the Pose of the Hare was the most comfortable at this time, and it also allowed my husband Phill easy access to my lower back for some firm massage.

At 9.00 my waters broke and I hopped into a warm bath. It was a very relaxing atmosphere with the warm water, candlelight, soft music and the gentle smell of Lavender. I hardly noticed the contractions while I was in the bath and I concentrated on slow deep breathing, counting steadily while breathing in and breathing out. I honestly could have stayed there all night, and when I did get out I felt like a new person, so calm and content. The thing that helped my backache and gave me the most relief when I got out of the bath was Phill tapping very firmly on my lower back, again in the Pose of the Hare

We arrived at the hospital at 10.30, and although I had to spend most of the time on my back for the midwife to monitor Morgan's heart beat, I concentrated on my breathing and my 'special place' Fleays, and stayed focused during the contractions. This took my mind off the pain while Phill continued to massage my back until I started to push. Having spent time in my 'special place' that afternoon was a fantastic help, not only was it fresh in my mind and much easier to imagine, but also because Phill was helping me to visualise by

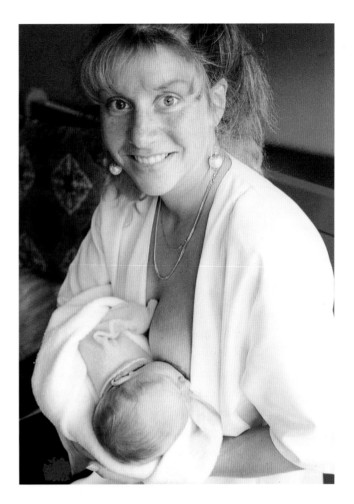

talking about the animals we had seen on our walk. Also the image of my baby in my arms seemed to make everything worthwhile and it also put the time frame into perspective, when I thought of how long I had waited for this moment in my life, it seemed reasonable to wait a few hours more.

With the CTG monitor still attached I rested in the Pose of the Hare in between contractions, and leant on the back of the bed on all fours to push, with gravity helping me. I found it really easy to push from this position and after Julie the midwife felt the head descending, she suggested bringing a mirror so I could watch the birth, which I thought was a fantastic idea. With my back against the raised bed, I had a perfect view and seeing Morgan's head appearing was unbelievably motivating. First a little grey spot, then Phill said, 'I can see hair'. I reached down and felt his head — it was

hard to believe I was actually touching my baby!!

At 2.05 a.m., out tumbled Morgan. From my angle all I saw was two legs and testicles!! 'It's a boy!' It was the most wonderful, most amazing thing I have ever experienced. Words cannot express my feelings.

I can't wait to do it again!!

Author's note: A very proud and elated Lindsay bought tiny Morgan back to the yoga class when he was just five days old, to show all the other pregnant mums to be. It was very encouraging for the other women to see Morgan and Lindsay so soon after the birth, especially as they were all first time mums. It was also very helpful for them to hear how her labour and birth had gone, especially as she had enjoyed it so much and had used the yoga breathing, visualisation techniques and some yoga positions to great benefit during labour.

7. Ebony Jade and Luke

I first became interested in yoga about eight years ago, after realising the benefits yoga can bring, physically, mentally, emotionally and spiritually, and I practised daily through both my pregnancies.

The squatting postures like The Salute and The Squat and Rise Pose [Gas Relieving Posture] were wonderful, as were the Pelvic Floor exercises for toning. I really loved lying on the floor with my legs up against the wall, as it stretched deeply into my hamstring muscles and made my legs feel strong, as did bending forward from the Wide-A Leg Stretch. I really appreciated the extra strength during labour, as I gave birth both times in a squatting position and both times my legs felt really strong. I practised all the other gentle yoga asanas that I enjoyed doing,

especially the easy Spinal Twists, The Heavenly Stretch Pose, The Triangle Poses and the Pelvic Tilt. I also practised the modified version of Salute To The Sun until I felt I was too big to continue.

I particularly enjoyed lying in the Flapping Fish Pose when I was feeling really big in the tummy, as I found it very comfortable for relaxation and tuning inwards to be with my baby. The breathing exercises I found the most useful were yogamudrasana, [The Psychic Union

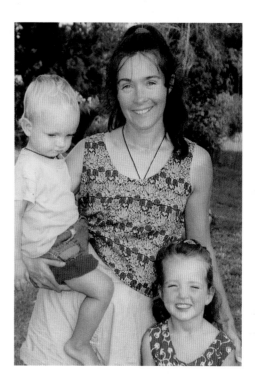

mudra] where the body slowly rocks forward and back, the Cooling Breath and the Alternate Nostril Breathing. I also loved doing the Humming Breath and felt the warm vibrations going to my baby.

My first labour with Ebony was a home birth. When I went into the labour, we discovered she was shoulder dystotia, which meant she was stuck by the shoulder behind my pubic bone. This meant a lot more pushing and a lot more time to move her beyond this point. I used a lot of slow, deep breathing throughout the labour which I felt helped me immensely as progress was very slow. After a 25 hour labour, 13 hours of that being

The complete book of
yoga and meditation
for pregnancy

second stage, Ebony Jade was finally born, 9 lb and a beautiful little angel. I never expected the birth to be like it was, but there are no rules with birth and you just don't know until you get there.

Luke's birth was much easier, lasting 8 hours and fairly smooth. I spent a lot of time in a warm bath in the Cat Pose and the water definitely helped soothe the pain. The second stage was only one hour long, but still incredibly intense. Those last, final pushes where Luke's head and body were delivered were quite amazing. I remember feeling the bulge of his head between my legs and the total strength it took to achieve that, and then the relief on the final push when his whole body followed. Luke was 8 lb 10 oz, and a gentle soul.

When I look back on the birth of my two children, I feel warm and fond feelings for the whole experience. Once the moment it is over, it's hard to recall the pain and discomfort, and of course we have the joy of our baby in our arms. Pregnancy has been the healthiest time in my life and it put me in such a mellow space, which was complemented by yoga. I found by practising 30 minutes each day I became really toned up and it helped me to stay focused throughout the whole pregnancy and birth.

8. Birthing and yoga: Sharman Okan's story

I have always been convinced that the female body knows, innately, how to give birth and so any process that helps to awaken, or tune into, that natural potential ought to be as widely advocated as possible. Yoga, for me, is one of the most compatible of these natural modalities for assisting the body, mind, emotions and spirit to birth gracefully, and in harmony with nature.

I have two children and two completely different birth stories. When

first pregnant with my daughter Lo-Arna, my long time partner departed the relationship for greener pastures. I spent the entire pregnancy and most of the first year of my daughter's life emotionally devastated. The one thing I kept returning to, for some kind of balance, was my yoga practise, which became my solace and my source of regeneration. From the age of 17 to 28 I had lived in a yoga Ashram as a Swami, studying and practising many techniques of yoga as a way of life. This

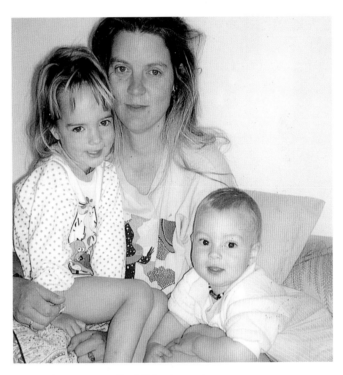

was what I naturally fell back on, during pregnancy, as a means to stay in touch with the greater picture, the universal quality of the experience of gestation and birth. Yoga helped me keep some kind of equilibrium so I did not get swamped in the emotional desolation of my situation.

I gave birth to Lo-Arna at home with a midwife and a couple of close friends. In retrospect, I see that the postpartum haemorrhage I suffered was emotionally precipitated due to the extent of the grief I had been experiencing. However, I did manage to give birth successfully in isolated conditions and, during the recovery from loss of blood, it *was solely my understanding of yogic breath awareness which got me through the ordeal. I think it probably saved my life actually and I did not lose consciousness at all, even though my blood pressure fell to an alarming 40/0! It was only my 'second nature' ability to focus, unwavered, on my incoming and outgoing breath, that kept me from going through the tunnel of death into the light at the other end, which I could see beckoning me. My midwife was incredible during all of this and supported me and tiny Lo-Arna through a hairy ride, from my mountain-top home to hospital.*

I would never have thought, at the time of this fateful dash into the arms of a recriminating faction of the medical profession, that less than three years hence, I would be giving birth again, to my son, Jevaan, in a hospital! However, give birth I did under completely different and happier circumstances. My midwife and dear friend, Pip, was once again with me, in the country town hospital of Murwillumbah, to help Jevaan into the world. She was as pregnant as I was, which was why we had opted for hospital. The midwives at the hospital were brilliant and greatly restored my appreciation of the best of the medical profession. My beloved partner Guy, Jenaan's father, was a tower of gentle strength and love, and the whole experience was a great healing for me. During my second pregnancy and birth I didn't need to use my yogic knowledge to just survive – I had the joy of performing the wonderful postures, breathing, relaxation and meditation techniques to have an easy, harmonious and transcendental experience of growing and birthing my son.

I cannot imagine ever approaching birth – indeed life and death, without the illumination of yoga.

9. Sandra's story. The birth of Jessie Ry Stevens

I began practising yoga during my first pregnancy when I was about 26 weeks and continued going to the classes weekly until I was well and truly due. I loved the squatting exercises because they felt so good as well as the breathing, and especially enjoyed the meditations and visualisations. I felt I was learning skills that would enable me to be more in control and that I could take into the labour with me. Having practised the various breathing and visualisation techniques during my pregnancy, I was therefore prepared when I finally went

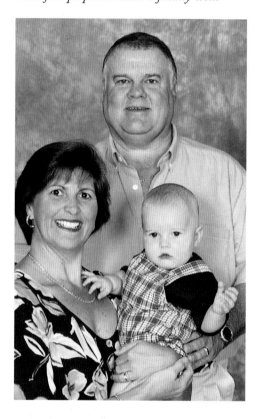

into labour. The skills I had learnt all came back to me so easily. When I closed my eyes I was totally centred on myself and the process of labour and I was able to be at peace with myself. Even though I had the support of Jake and the hospital staff, when you are in labour you are really on your own and it was at this time that the visualisation of colour was such a great advantage.

186

The complete book of
yoga and meditation
for pregnancy
∞

After visiting the doctor on Wednesday at lunch time, I prepared myself for the birth of my baby the following day. The doctor said I was 2 cm dilated and that although the head was not engaged, as this was an IVF pregnancy he would put me into hospital that night. Gel would be inserted at midnight and if labour had not started by early the following morning, he would rupture my membranes.

So, we went off to Allamanda Hospital at 7.30 p.m. along with my yoga info and poses, antenatal books, massage oils, music, etc.; and with a birth plan floating around in my head. My husband and I had discussed what we wanted to do, walking, squatting, breathing, massage . . . I was preparing myself mentally for a long day of moving around in labour.

At 11.30 p.m. when I was first connected to the CTG monitor, I was feeling some contractions, albeit like slight period pains. The gel was then inserted and about one and a half hours later, I was really feeling what the monitor was indicating. I was left to get some sleep but was awakened regularly every 9 or 10 minutes with more pain. I kept trying to sleep, still thinking this was going to go on all night and into the next day. By 2.30 a.m. I was up and walking around, feeling a little uncomfortable, and once I had a show I was confident to call the nurses in for assistance.

By 3 a.m. the nurses decided that we had better phone my husband and to move into the delivery room. 'Already!' I thought. Jake arrived a little later but we were told I would be a long time yet. However, my waters broke and I was full-on into labour, it was all happening so fast that the tapes, massage oils and other accessories I wanted to use were in the corner of the room unused. However, I used the controlled deep yoga breathing which I felt was really helpful and I

visualised my baby moving down through the birth canal as I did this breathing. With the help of a little gas, it was a marvellous experience and I found it all so easy, while the breathing helped me to stay focused and able to cope. Jake's role was to keep me cool with wet washes and an aromatherapy atomiser occasionally sprayed onto my face. At 5 a.m. my doctor was called in and with a lot of pushing and encouragement our son, Jessie Ry Stevens was born at 5.35 that Thursday morning.

We forgot to ask the staff to lower the mirror so that we could both witness the birth. However, using visualisation techniques I had learned in yoga classes, I visualised his entry into this world. I felt like I'd seen my son long before I laid eyes on him for real, during some meditations I had done in yoga. It was quite a powerful feeling. Jessie weighed 8 lb 3 oz, and I required 3 stitches, but all was well.

We had our son!

10. Jera Conan

I was 35, pregnant for the first time and in a state of shock! Fortunately, I had 15 years of yoga experience within me to help and the same amount of years teaching yoga, including (luckily) antenatal courses. Through these classes I had become aware that each pregnancy and birth was distinct and that, with time and practise, each woman intuitively chose different yoga practices for her particular needs and focus. The important thing seemed to be knowing a variety of postures, pranayama, relaxation and meditation techniques in order to keep up with one's changing body and feelings, thereby enabling the spontaneous choice of what practice to use at any time. I was now to prove this for myself over the next 9 months!

Throughout the first 4 months I continued most asanas and pranayama I'd

187

Birth
Birth journeys

always used, adding more butterfly and squats, yoga nidra relaxation and accenting Om chanting meditation. As soon as I felt uncomfortable with any posture I stopped it (or in some cases adapted it) and gradually simplified the breathing practices so I always felt at ease with my breath. I had very little physical

discomfort throughout my pregnancy and feel that this was because of my daily practice of asanas, a knowledge of how to relax when I became tired or tense and a healthy vegetarian diet.

I was lucky enough to have a home birth with both doctor and midwife who advocated yoga. My labour was about 10 hours. During a lot of this time my awareness automatically went to my natural breath. I rarely consciously changed my breathing patterns (unless directed to), simply followed the spontaneous changes that naturally occurred throughout. I could not have

done this had I not regularly practised the different pranayamas. As well as physically helping with pain and giving energy, breath awareness became my source of balance and focus.

After Leuke was born I needed these yoga practices even more! - to learn about my 'new' baby yet again, cope with 'new' feelings (help!) and to go patiently with myself so as not to be overwhelmed with being a mother. I made myself continue straight away with a very shortened, simple version of what I'd been doing in my last months of pregnancy, gradually adding more as I felt possible. Leuke is now 8 and yoga remains at the centre of my life, especially as a mother, just as in those first 9 months of pregnancy.

11. Jessica Reilly: Pregnancy, birth and yoga

I decided to begin yoga classes during the second trimester of my pregnancy. It was to be the first time I had tried yoga and my first experiences were at my gym, which held yoga classes a few times a week. The instructors were very good, however, as my pregnancy progressed, the moves were becoming more difficult. The instructors would show me alternative moves to the remainder of the class, which would be more suited to my requirements. It was at that time I was due to visit the maternity unit again, and found that Theresa was conducting yoga classes specifically catering for pregnant women. I decided to try these classes and see how they differed from those at the gym.

Why did I decide to try yoga classes during pregnancy?

There were a number of reasons for this decision. Firstly, my husband was trying to get me to learn to relax after years of stress, poor eating habits and lack of exercise while I was working as a

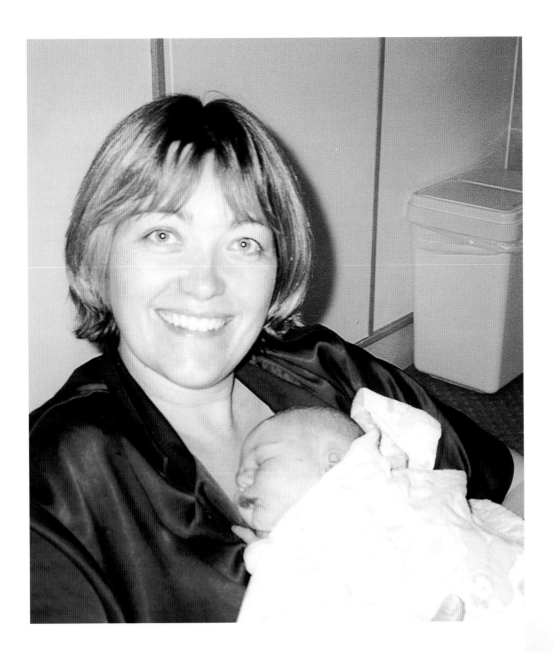

Pharmaceutical Sales Representative and then another short stint back in the classroom in my previous role of a Secondary Science Teacher. I found it difficult to relax and would often find myself clenching my teeth as I slept. I was also taking short rapid breaths while sleeping, and waking up in the morning not feeling refreshed from sleep, even though I may have slept for 7-8 hours. I realised that for my own sake and also my unborn child's I really needed to rectify this problem. The solution was to try yoga to learn to relax and breathe correctly. There was an added benefit in the stretching exercises, which helped to

improve my suppleness in preparation for the birth. This led me to Theresa's classes.

These classes differed from those at the gym in that the exercises and breathing techniques were all aimed at the pregnant woman and her requirements. I found them much easier and finally felt I had found somewhere, which would help me learn to breathe correctly, not only for the birth, but also for life. The classes would begin with stretching exercises, and move onto the breathing and meditation exercises. I think we all found these wonderful, and I am sure we all managed to drop off to sleep on more than one occasion!

The result!

My breathing improved, I found myself more relaxed and my husband told me that my breathing at night was much better. I was actually starting to feel as though I had a good night's sleep (as much as you can when you are entering the final stages of pregnancy!) I found that the meditations were the best. My particular favourite was the candle meditation, which would relax me almost instantly and I also found it the easiest to focus on. The meditations involving choosing a colour and a 'place' were also very good and they did help while I was in labour, which leads me onto the next aspect, how did yoga help me?

I went into labour on a Sunday afternoon and had to go to hospital immediately as my waters had broken. I did not use any pain relief at all through the afternoon and night. I was very focused on what I was doing and also used the different breathing techniques I was shown to help me through the contractions as they increased in intensity (antenatal classes so not teach breathing techniques anymore). My husband and I attended the partners' evening where he was shown some of the breathing and meditation techniques I had been learning. This proved very beneficial as he helped me (reminded me) what I had learnt and encouraged me to use those breathing techniques. It was unfortunate that the candle could not be used in the labour ward (no open flames are permitted in the hospital rooms), but I did focus on a light, which helped. At 6 a.m. the following morning, I began on the gas, as the contractions were becoming much more intense. One and a half hours later there was bedlam in the room as my son was in distress and we had to have an emergency caesarean with a general anaesthetic. I awoke to a very healthy young boy whom we called Loughlin Thomas Reilly.

Loughlin is a very placid and relaxed child. I feel within myself that part of this is because I learnt to relax with the yoga classes during my pregnancy (I continued them until the week I had Loughlin), and I am still using the basic techniques I learnt whenever I become uptight again. There was another bonus to these classes. I met a number of wonderful ladies whom I am still in contact with. We meet on a regular basis and continue the friendship that was begun in the classes. I there was another bonus to these classes it was that we had an avenue to discuss our pregnancy and ventilate our feelings with a group of people who were also going through the same changes in their lives. It was a wonderful support network and I would highly recommend it to any pregnancy woman!

The complete book of
yoga and meditation
for pregnancy

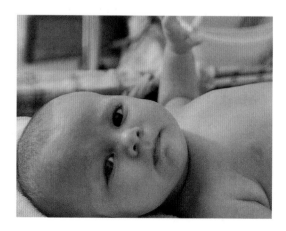

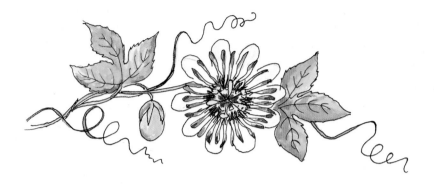

Important Skills for Labour

It is not possible to actually rehearse labour or really know what will happen. However, I feel that if you are well prepared your time during labour has to be better than if you went into it completely unprepared. When the time comes for labour to begin, there are a few valuable skills to remember, so you can move through the birthing process as gently and easily as possible.

When you are focused and centred in yourself – with the knowledge that you have prepared for this time mentally, emotionally and physically – you will have the self trust, inner strength and confidence to approach labour with a clear mind and a positive attitude. You will also be able to utilise all your physical strength and mental energies to be actively involved in the different stages of the birthing process with a one pointed awareness and sense of purpose. Even if you

encounter complications during the labour and things don't go exactly as planned – for example having a caesarean delivery when a natural birth was planned – the various skills you have learnt through your yoga practices will still prove to be of great benefit and support.

You will be familiar with most of the suggestions recommended here, from reading the various chapters in this book. I have also included some other suggestions which are not strictly connected with yoga but which have proven to be valuable aids to use for an easier and more comfortable delivery.

All of the following techniques are best used between contractions. Use those wonderful spaces to become still, centred and relaxed, and to recover from one contraction and prepare for the next one. For example, when one contraction has finished, relax in the most comfortable position, moving your awareness inwards, while visualising the energy within your breath restoring and replenishing your whole being with *prana*. Quietly talk to your baby and affirm all is well and that you are both doing fine. Maybe visualise yourself and your baby surrounded by a beautiful healing colour, glowing and radiant. Close your eyes and feel your breath moving deeply into your body, meditating and focusing on the healing power of each breath.

I feel it is very important to accept that there is always an element of uncertainty with labour. It cannot really be planned or controlled, unless you have a scheduled caesarean delivery. I have known a number of women who have been overwhelmed with disappointment when their natural birth didn't eventuate or they had to rely on analgesics instead of managing a drug free birth. This disappointment can sometimes lead to bonding and feeding problems and a detachment from the fact that they have just given birth to a beautiful, healthy baby. It's crucial to know where your focus is – even when you plan for an easy and natural delivery – so that you have an open mind and an attitude of acceptance.

In the end, what is most important is that both you and your baby are well and healthy, that you can enjoy this time in your life, acknowledge the wonder of being a woman and the miracle of birth, and trust in your inherent 'female wisdom' to move with the birthing process.

Breathing exercises & visualisations

Prepare yourself for labour by being familiar with your favourite breathing exercises and visualisation techniques. Always choose the practices that gave you the most benefits during pregnancy as they will give you the best opportunity to work deeply with your

body and the amazing energy of birth.

The energy of labour can sometimes take women by surprise and carry them far beyond what feels safe. Some women feel that an unknown 'greater' part of themselves emerges during labour. They come to know and experience the wonder and miracle of giving birth and of life itself. By utilising your breath and its energy, you will remain completely aware of the moment, staying clearly focused and able to use all of your own natural wisdom. In this way, you will move confidently with the labour rather than struggling against it which often causes fear and tension and increases the possibility of problems. The principle is the same as having your bag packed ready for hospital, only with these skills and suggestions you are well prepared mentally and spiritually with all the information you need ready for use in your mind

When practising the breathing exercises, keep in mind that the incoming breath will supply you with *prana* (energy) and all that you need to maintain balance and harmony in your body, mind and spirit. The outgoing breath can be used to release tension, anxiety and stress. The breathing practices are most valuable when used between contractions, so as to replenish lost physical energies, to restore emotional balance and mental clarity, and to prepare you for the next contraction.

The breathing exercises I have found to be the most useful during labour are: the Cooling Breath, *ujjayi pranayama* (the Breath of Tranquillity), the Complete Breath, the Cleansing Breath and the Humming Breath.

When practising the Cooling Breath, visualise a peaceful and calming place in nature, maybe somewhere you go often or a place you would love to visit, and 'draw' that image into your mind as the breath comes into your body. This concept is also very helpful when visualising a healing colour, to enhance the feelings most needed at the time. If you like to use colour in your visualisations, imagine the colour being drawn into your body with your breath, either to a specific part of your body, or around your whole body. Likewise, the result is equally beneficial when you focus on a word that will enhance the feelings most needed at the time, repeating the word to yourself each time you breathe in.

The *ujjayi pranayama* is especially good for turning your awareness inwards to where you become one with yourself and the whole breathing process. When the *ujjayi pranayama* is practised during labour, it will become aware of your body and of your baby, the quality of your thoughts and your emotional nature.

Labour and childbirth really are a time to be completely absorbed in all aspects of yourself and the process of labour, so it is helpful to communicate gently with your baby and imagine he or she moving easily through the birth canal. Placing your hands on your abdomen at this time will help you connect you with your baby, who I am sure will feel the warmth of your touch and sense the softness of your thoughts.

Ujjayi pranayama is particularly useful as you approach transition where you might begin to feel scattered and vague. It is also particularly valuable if your energies are diminishing during the second stage of labour. It can be practised in any position, either sitting up or lying down, with full deep breathing or continuously with the natural breath.

Deep Yoga Breathing is an extremely valuable exercise to use throughout labour as the incoming breath will replenish all the positive,

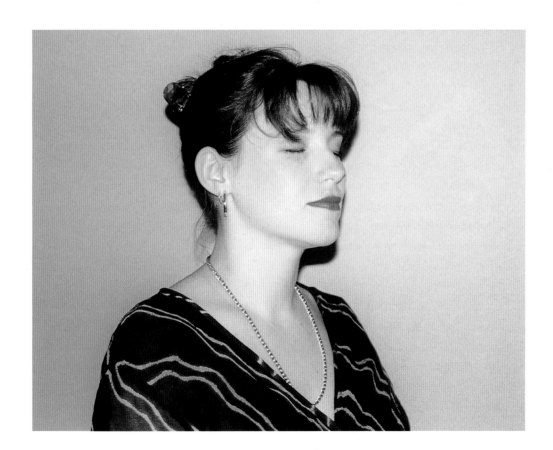

calming and energising qualities you will need, while the outgoing breath can release tensions on all levels thereby helping you to relax and become settled. When you are breathing deeply, you might like to visualise healing energy in the form of light or a particular colour creating the appropriate atmosphere in your body and mind. As this beautiful image of light fills the entire body and mind, all confusion, tension and anxiety are more easily removed.

The Cleansing Breath is excellent for releasing tension and stress on all levels, thereby helping to minimise and eliminate any anxiety or doubt. As you exhale strongly through your mouth, you will feel all tension and discomfort being blown out and away from your body and mind, leaving you relaxed and calm.

The Humming Breath enables you to tune in with your own healing sound. A number of women I know have used the Humming Breath during labour to help overcome pain, to stay focused in the present moment, and to increase their inner strength by adding the dimension of sound to their great effort. They found it extremely powerful to hum deeply through the more intense contractions of the later stages of labour, feeling and visualising the vibrations penetrating into the womb.

It really helps to make some noise during labour, and often it is a sound which most women have never heard themselves make yet at the same time is both familiar and extremely potent. When the time comes to increase the energy and strength required for childbirth the sound often heard is deep, primordial and ancient. It is a unique sound, characteristic to all women and one which connects them to each other. The Humming Breath resembles this deep feminine sound and

connects you with your inner self, often to a point where the sound seems to resonate through your body, deep into your soul where you can feel it and listen to it at the same time.

The Humming Breath will compose and centre your mind, while connecting you with an extraordinary stillness and peace deep inside, so valuable during labour. When the contractions begin to intensify, focus your awareness inwards and inhale slowly, drawing in all the *prana* and energy you will need. Breathe out and hum deeply while concentrating your whole awareness on moving the stored energy down into the birth canal. The combination of your breath, your total awareness and the humming sound will provide you with a valuable source of power and energy for going with the birthing process. I am sure your baby will also benefit from the healing sounds and vibrations.

Affirmations

The use of affirmations helps maintain the connection with yourself, your energies and your baby. There are many excellent books of affirmations, but sometimes it's better to compose your own as they will have a more personal feel than those thought out by someone else. If you wish to do this, always choose words that are positive, never using words such as fear, panic, anxiety or pain. This is especially relevant if you have had a previous pregnancy and birthing experience that was difficult in some way. It is important to concentrate on the present moment and to work with the positive energy available to you at the time, rather than reliving a past experience through fear, doubt and panic.

The affirmations can be said out loud, to yourself, or written down and

194

The complete book of
yoga and meditation
for pregnancy

read during the day. Some people find it very helpful to write their affirmations a number of times each day until they are comfortable with the feel of the words. In this way, the words can be changed until the affirmation is perfect for the situation.

Here are a few examples that could be used during pregnancy and labour. Remember to change the words if they don't feel right for you.

your affirmations so they can remind you of them during labour, especially if you become vague or disorientated at that time.

Father's affirmations

Sometimes the father of the baby will feel detached or disconnected from the whole pregnancy, for the simple reason that he is not carrying the baby and his view of things is quite different

---

I allow my whole being to embrace and flow with the natural process of labour.

I move easily and gently through the birthing process, my baby is born safely and in peace.

My body and mind express radiance and love. I am a beautiful woman.

I am calm, centred and at peace with myself, my pregnancy and becoming a mother.

I love being a woman, I embrace my pregnancy and I joyfully look forward to becoming a mother.

I welcome and accept the changes in my body and the new life growing inside me.

My child is welcome and loved, and I give thanks for the miracle of life.
I am truly blessed.

I gently and lovingly nurture myself and my baby. I am at peace.

I lovingly release my baby into the world. I am at peace with the miracle of birth.

I acknowledge the power of my body and nature, to assist me to give birth easily and gently.

I am safe, supported and loved, I move forward with peace and ease.

I love, accept and appreciate myself just how I am.
All is well in my world.

You are loved, you are special, you are welcome. (To the baby.)

The more these ideas and techniques are thought about and practised while you are pregnant, the easier it will be to bring them to mind during labour. There are other visualisations and meditations that are suitable to use during labour and for a more detailed study ask at specialised bookshops for literature on these subjects. It is also a good idea to encourage your partner and other birth support people to become familiar with

from the mother's. However, his role is of equal importance and significance, and it would be very appropriated if the father would create some affirmations of his own – just a few simple words of special relevance for him. These might be in reference to his role as a father and a parent or his deep inner feelings towards his baby. This will give him the opportunity to communicate and bond with his baby before the birth, just as the mother is doing.

A special place in nature

Over the years, I have noticed many women responding favourably to the concept of visualising a special place in nature, or a place that has particular relevance for them. The mere thought and image of this place will make you feel calm and safe, and this can be a very useful technique to remember during labour. When a woman chooses a beautiful and peaceful place from her own experiences or from her imagination, she can relate to it personally and become more completely involved. You might choose a place that

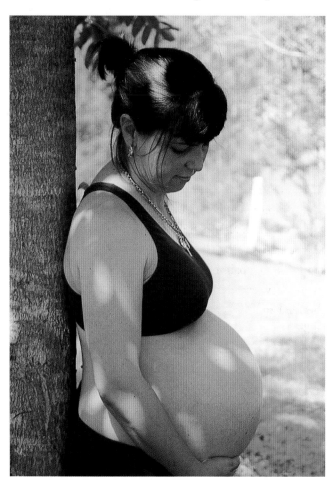

196

The complete book of
yoga and meditation
for pregnancy

is frequented often or a place from childhood or from your past. Some women prefer to visualise an imaginary place that has safe and pleasant feelings for them. The important thing to remember is to choose somewhere that will calm your mind and induce deeper states of relaxation, whether that place is imaginary or not.

In the chapter, 'Birth Journeys', Lindsay used this technique to great benefit during her labour. Whenever we did this meditation in class, she would always imagine she was in the nature reserve behind her home, which is a beautiful and serene place. When she was in the early moments of labour she went for a walk in the reserve with her husband to help stay calm and relaxed. Then, later on during the final stages of labour, she again focused on this special place and found it helped her stay composed and in the moment. It is a true example of bringing the world of imagery into the real world. Other women take a photo of their special place with them into the delivery suite.

The best way to use this idea is to sit quietly and relax for a few minutes. When you are calm and ready, bring to mind your special place. Let your imagination expand as you explore this place using all your senses to fully experience every aspect. Imagine the time of day or night you are there and the season of the year, as this will influence what you see and what you feel. Imagine the colours you see, the taste and smell of the air and the different textures and surfaces. Allow yourself to become completely involved in your own meditation and, most importantly, observe the feeling in your body and the atmosphere in your mind. For the best results, do this as often as you can before labour so that you will be able to bring your special place to mind when you most need it.

Colour

The concept of using colour during meditation appeals to many women. During labour it is often used to maintain balance, harmony and calmness. If you have found colour meditation beneficial during pregnancy, it will be a valuable tool for helping you to stay calm and relaxed when you are in labour. For more information on colour in meditation, refer to the chapter, 'Visualisation & Creative Meditations'.

Relaxation positions for labour

In the last few weeks of your pregnancy, spend some time resting in the relaxation positions you have found to be the most comfortable. Consider which ones you might like to use during labour. These might include the Pose of the Hare or the Flapping Fish. Some women find it very helpful to 'rehearse' for labour by resting in one of these positions, imagining they are between contractions and utilising the breathing techniques and visualisations. Always remember to use pillows or cushions – both while you are pregnant and during labour – to ensure complete comfort.

The candle meditation

It is not permitted to have a lit candle in a hospital, but you might find the candle meditation valuable in the early stages of labour when you are still at home. Of course, if you are having your baby at home there are no restrictions on what you choose to do.

If you are able to stay at home in early labour – and feel safe and comfortable with that – I suggest spending the time soaking in a lovely warm bath with a little lavender oil and the candle flame in a position that is easy for you to see. With the atmosphere created, you can relax in the warm water and be calmed by the

lavender aroma while gazing at the brightest point of the flame. You might even like to have your favourite music playing in the background.

This might all sound a bit far-fetched when you are trying to cope with being in labour, but I have known women who have done exactly this, finding it a very suitable way to stay calm and to prepare for the more involved part of labour.

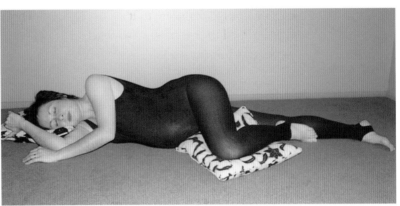

Handling pain during labour

Everybody has a different pain threshold and, although you may have encountered pain at other times during your life, the pain of labour can be a whole new experience. I am a little hesitant to use the word 'pain' when talking about labour and childbirth, as it immediately creates tension and unpleasant images or memories. I prefer instead to refer to the intense physical feelings you will experience during labour, and to discuss the management of those feelings. The more centred, relaxed and in command of your emotions and thoughts you can be during labour, the better you will manage the discomfort.

By 'going with' the strain or physical stress you are feeling – in contrast to trying to ignore it, which is difficult – the easier it will be to handle and the more it will appear to mellow and soften. When your attention is held firmly in the present moment and you are completely absorbed by your breathing or your body, the more gently you will merge with the whole experience.

Some women feel it very helpful to 'colour' the intense feelings. Firstly concentrate on the feelings, and then surround them with a healing colour so as to soften and disperse them with your imagination. Spend some time before your due date thinking about what might be the most useful and helpful for you, so when the time comes you are prepared and ready.

Bach Flower and Australian Bush Flower remedies

I feel it relevant to mention the use of English Bach Flower and Australian Bush Flower remedies for pregnancy, and especially during labour. Their subtle yet profound qualities balance and calm the emotions. For the most beneficial results it is appropriate to consult a qualified practitioner rather then choosing a remedy for yourself. The flower essences work on the emotional body and are best made up to suit your personal needs at a specific time.

These remedies are safe to use during times of mental and emotional stress, indecision and confusion. I feel it is very important to point out that vibrational medicines will not fix or solve an emotional problem or issue. However, they do seem to soften the heightened emotions around the issue. When our energy changes around a problem and we see it in another light, solutions can more easily be found.

During labour these remedies will gently relax you, easing your mind and emotions so you are able to stay with what is happening rather than becoming confused, fearful or disorientated. During pregnancy, they are a non-invasive way of managing the various emotional changes that naturally occur. I personally found the Bach Flowers very suitable after birth, as they helped me move through the massive hormonal and emotional changes that occurred, without experiencing the after birth 'blues'. If a more severe depression occurs after the birth, they can be used in combination with other important therapies. The remedies will also come to the 'rescue' if you are emotionally troubled while breastfeeding, as your frame of mind will cause changes in your body's chemistry and therefore affect your breast milk. Even if you are not breastfeeding, your baby will instinctively know when you are upset.

Music

Some women feel it is comforting to have a favourite piece of soft music playing in the background during labour, to soothe and relax them. During your pregnancy it is a good idea to become familiar with one or two special pieces of music that have a calming effect on your mind and body so that during labour the sound of that music will relax you.

Essential Oils

There are a number of beautiful essential oils that are safe to use during pregnancy and labour. Care needs to be taken when choosing oils because some are toxic and can cause premature labour.

The best oils for pregnancy are Lavender, Rose, Rosewood, Ylang Ylang, Mandarin, Geranium, Sandalwood, Lemon, Frankincense, Petitgrain and Neroli.

Caution: Always avoid the following essential oils during pregnancy: Basil, Cedarwood, Cinnamon, Camphor, Chamomile, Juniper, Fennel, Hyssop, Marjoram, Melissa, Myrrh, Pennyroyal, Sage, Rosemary and Thyme.

The recommended oils can be used as massage oils or in a bath where no more than nine drops are added. Some women like to be massaged during labour, especially on the abdomen, lower back, shoulders, feet and legs. Others prefer not to be touched at all, but receive wonderful benefits from rubbing the oils lightly into their temples. The Pose of the Hare is an ideal posture to rest in for a soothing massage, especially when the lower back area is uncomfortable during labour.

The best oils for labour are Lavender and Jasmine, which can be used together or on their own. Lavender is well known as a relaxing herb, useful for treating mild anxiety, insomnia and nervous tension. Lavender will assist in balancing the whole person and, when used with other relaxation techniques and breathing exercises, will prove to be invaluable during labour. Jasmine is a uterine tonic and will assist with the contractions, while it is also an important essential oil for anxiety, depression and pain management. Jasmine is also a beautiful oil to use after the birth if there is any depression or if you are feeling 'low'. Clary-sage is another oil recommended for the final stages of labour. It is a uterine tonic and has been known to assist pain relief and to encourage uterine contractions. All these oils should be used in a 1 to 2 percent dilution and are best added to a good quality base oil such as cold pressed almond oil or avocado oil.

When you pack your bag for the hospital, remember to take a bottle of the relevant essential oils with you to help maintain balance and calmness during labour, and relaxation after the delivery. However, for the specialised needs of pregnancy and labour, consult a qualified aromatherapist who will mix the relevant oils for you.

It is my hope that you find the suggestions and recommendations detailed here valuable and of real benefit during pregnancy and childbirth, and that your labour be as calm and gentle as possible.

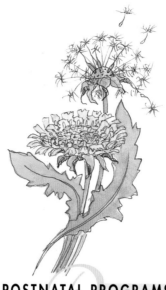

POSTNATAL PROGRAMS
Birth to Six Months

Postnatal

The first six weeks

After the birth of your baby, your time and attention will be involved with caring for your newborn and exploring the joy and wonder of being a mother. If this is your first child, you will be discovering what a full-time job motherhood is, and how little time there seems to be for anything else, particularly in the first few months. In the early days of your baby's life, close bonds and spiritual relationships are formed between you, your child and your partner, which last a lifetime. During this time, you will come to know your baby's unique personality. Motherhood is one of life's most precious gifts, and these early days need to be cherished and savoured as they disappear all too quickly. It is well worth allowing the time to be fully absorbed by these brief moments in your life and catching up on the rest of life at some time in the future.

During these early days of caring for your new baby, it is very important to make sure your own needs are not being neglected. Have plenty of rest, eat nourishing foods and drink plenty of fluids, especially if you are breastfeeding. For many women this is an exhausting time and there seems to be no space left for rest and relaxation.

Many women who have practised yoga during their pregnancies have commented on how valuable the various skills were after the birth. It is not advised that you begin exercises or postures until after the lochia (after birth bleeding) has completely ceased. However, this is an ideal time to resume deep relaxation, breathing exercises and meditation. These can be continued as soon after the birth as you wish. They will assist in restoring balance and harmony on all levels, and will help to replenish your energies. I also strongly advise continuation of the pelvic floor

200

The complete book of
yoga and meditation
for pregnancy

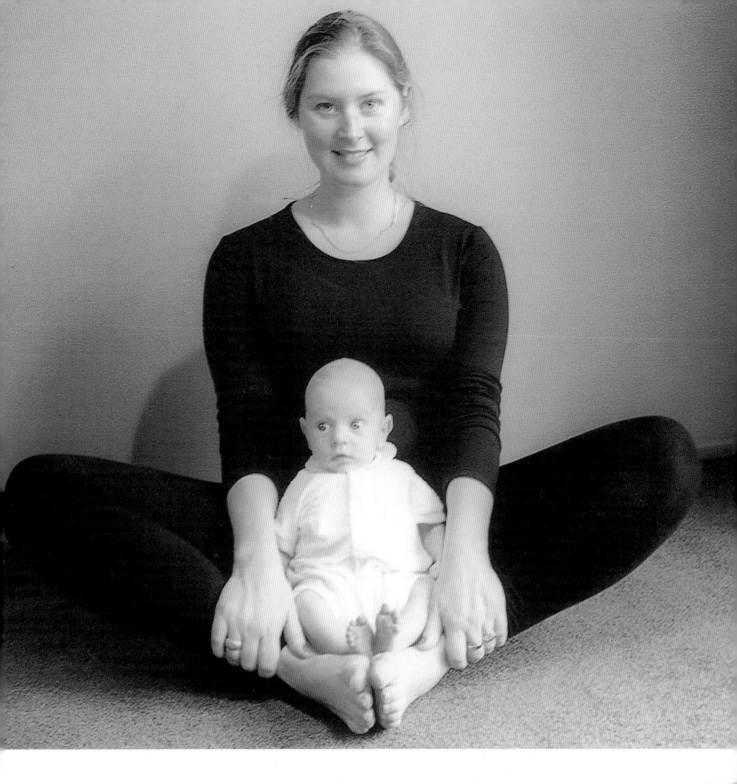

exercises soon after the birth, to return firmness and strength to your perineum and pelvic floor muscles.

If the birth was reasonably straightforward, it is also quite acceptable to include a few gentle head lifts, to restore tone and fitness to your abdominal area. These are best done from a lying position with your knees bent. Practise slowly and without effort, up to nine times each day. However, more time is needed for recovery if you

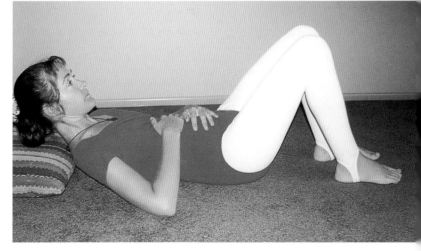

had an exhausting labour or a caesarean delivery and as a general rule always ask your doctor or midwife before proceeding with these exercises.

Most importantly, relax as often as possible and continue with all the breathing exercises. Any stretching exercises should be avoided until at least four to six weeks after the birth, and fitness programs or strenuous exercises should be postponed until your baby is a lot older.

The postnatal exercise and yoga program detailed here will not be suitable for every woman, as your wellbeing, the health of your baby and your baby's temperament will all have a bearing on whether you are ready – or even interested – in doing yoga again so soon after the birth. If you are having an easy time feeding your baby and your baby has settled well, you will be more likely to consider doing some gentle exercises than if your baby has colic and your sleep pattern is completely disturbed.

My intention here is to outline a well balanced and easy to manage program which can be integrated into your daily activities by spending a little time whenever it is appropriate for you in the comfort of your own home. Many of the exercises recommended can even be done while watching TV or sitting in your garden under a shady tree with your baby.

Remember not to be too strict or obsessive with yourself when contemplating an exercise program after the birth. Your body has just undergone some massive changes physically and emotionally, and your hormones are adjusting again. Be gentle with yourself and realise that you will regain your shape and figure over time. Don't panic when your favourite clothes don't fit in the first weeks and even months after

the birth. It is a fact of life that some women seem to return to their pre-pregnancy shape more quickly than others, but that's because we are all unique and are made so differently.

Six weeks after the birth

When your baby is 5 or 6 weeks old you may feel it is the right time to begin some gentle yoga exercises. The exercises recommended will restore tone and flexibility, and remove any stiffness you might be feeling. Approach your yoga with a quite mind and gentle attitude. You will be happier and more relaxed, and this state of being will help your baby to stay calm and relaxed too.

There are many benefits to be gained from resuming a simple yoga and exercises program after the birth. Your pelvic floor muscles and your perineum are encouraged to become firm and strong. The muscles of your uterus are assisted in returning to normal size. Your back is kept supple and flexible, while your spinal column and your spinal nerves are nourished and strengthened. This will help to relieve any tension held in your neck and back muscles. Your abdominal muscles are firmed and toned and your circulation is improved and maintained. Fatigue is managed better and energy levels improved. Relaxation and nervous stability are encouraged, especially when breathing exercises, meditation and relaxation practices are included. Your tolerance and patience will increase and you will survive lack of sleep better.

Caution: At no time are the exercises meant to cause strain or result in fatigue. Begin slowly with the simpler stretches and postures and approach them in such a way as to nurture and fulfill your needs rather than as a work-out program!

202

The complete book of
yoga and meditation
for pregnancy

1. Choose a selection of exercises and postures from the chapter, ëWarming Up'. All the exercises in that chapter are gentle and easy to do. For example, one day do the Hand and Feet exercises and other corresponding exercises, maybe the Butterfly, the Shoulder exercises, a little pranayama and some deep relaxation.

2. On another day, warm your body first and then practise the Head and Neck exercises, the Eye exercises, followed by the Pelvic Floor exercises, the Hamstring Stretch, the Cat and the Tiger.

3. If you enjoyed the balancing postures, I would also add the Tree and an easy Spinal Twist to your selection. Whatever you choose to do, always start by loosening your body first, and finish with some breathing exercises and deep relaxation.

4. This gentle program will take no more than 15 minutes at the most to complete.

Eight to twelve weeks after the birth

If you feeling well and strong around 8 to 12 weeks after the birth, you might like to add the following postures to your routine. Before continuing on with any more postures, however, obtain your doctor's approval.

The yoga postures can be approached almost as a meditation in motion, feeling yourself moving from one position to the next as the breath is unified with the movements and you witness your inner self and the flow of energy (*prana*) deep within you. You will notice a profound sense of grace and stillness when yoga is practised in this way.

1. The Intense Forward Stretch

Do this with your feet a little apart and when returning to the standing position bend your knees slightly to guard against straining your back.

2. The Mountain

Rest into the Pose of the Child from time to time to gain relief from this strong posture.

3. The Heavenly Stretch

4. The Easy Seated Spinal Twist

The Waist Rotation and spinal twist exercise is also suitable.

5. The Deep Standing Squat

This deep standing squat builds strength and endurance by working strongly into your hips, buttocks and thigh muscles.

6. Triangle Side Bend

By completing a forward bend, a spinal twist and a side bend, you are working the spinal column in most directions giving your back more flexibility. All of these exercises are simple and safe to do unless you are experiencing back problems or have been advised by a professional not to do them.

7. The Single Leg Lifts lying on your back

These are done in exactly the same way as they were done during pregnancy. These exercises are excellent for toning your abdominal muscles. The abdominal muscles take time and patience to regain their original firmness after pregnancy and birth. When practising these leg exercises, always have one leg slightly bent with your foot on the floor, as the other leg is lifted.

At no time continue with these exercises if the abdominal area becomes ëshaky', or if your breathing becomes short and tense. These are signs of straining beyond your limits. Flatten the middle of your back by pressing it to the floor, so you are using your abdominal muscles rather than your back muscles to lift your leg. This is also a safeguard against straining your back. Some women find it helpful to place their hands – palms down – under their hips when practising the leg lifts and any of the other abdominal exercises, as it encourages the back to stay flat on the floor instead of arching.

Twelve weeks after the birth

When your baby is around 12 weeks old, your life will have settled considerably and you might have more energy and a little more time. At this time you can add the following exercises to those you are already practising, again choosing a few from each section to make a complete mini yoga program of your own. Choose the postures that suit your personal needs, remembering to enjoy them.

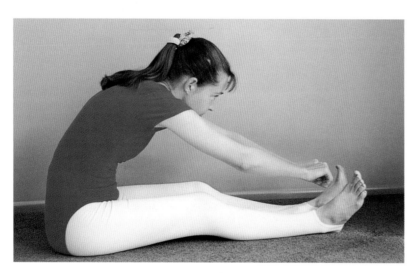

These yoga exercises are a general guideline for you to follow while ever they are helping you and are making you feel good. Always listen to your body and do what is best for you, moving along slowly and quietly at your own pace. The dangers of not listening to your body and of ignoring early warnings such as painful muscles and

fatigue could, over time, lead to a decreased milk supply, sleep disorders or emotional problems such as moodiness, depression and irritability. When the body's signals are completely ignored, it becomes exhausted and more serious conditions can develop.

The yoga postures can be approached almost as a meditation in motion, feeling yourself moving from one posture to the next as your breath and your movements are unified – always witnessing your inner self and the flow of energy and *prana* deep within you. You will notice a profound sense of grace and stillness when yoga is practised in this way.

Remember to allow time to include breathing exercises, meditation and relaxation techniques. To begin with, you might only have time to do one or two postures at a time, but this is still very beneficial and certainly better than not doing any at all. Now you can also include the other balancing and triangle postures. This is quite an adequate group of postures and, unless you have a personal desire or need to do something more strenuous and demanding, I would continue on as detailed until your baby is at least 6 months old.

1. Rowing the Boat

Now that you are not pregnant, you can extend back much further than you were able to during pregnancy. This means you will now be working more deeply into your abdominal area. Do not lean right back to the floor but recline enough to feel your abdominal muscles working. If you go too close to the floor, returning to the upright position can strain your lower back muscles.

The complete book of yoga and meditation for pregnancy

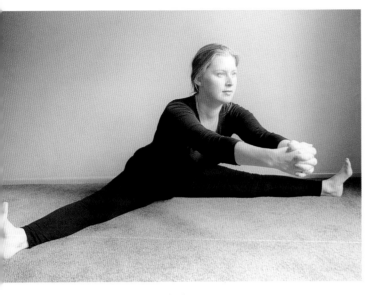

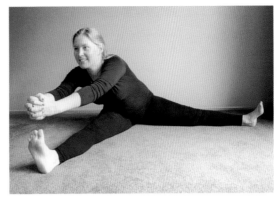

straight and your other leg bent (Head to Knee posture), but now it can be done with both legs straight. You will be aware of a much deeper stretch throughout the muscles of your back and the hamstrings at the back of your legs, and care needs to be taken not to overextend or force yourself into the final posture. The benefits are similar for both postures, only to a greater degree in this one. It is highly recommended for women who suffer menstrual difficulties and is an ideal postnatal exercise. However, it is not suitable for people who have severe back problems such as slipped discs. Always rest in the Pose of the Child when you have completed the posture.

2. Churning the Mill

The same principles apply for this posture as the previous one, as you can now take your body further back towards the floor. Again, this works much more deeply into your abdominal muscles.

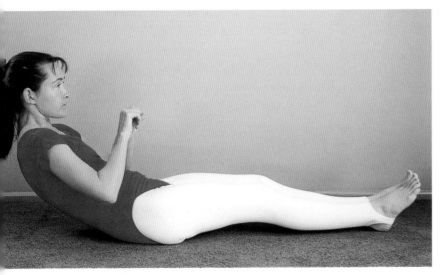

Top left: Churning the Mill
Left: Rowing the Boat

3. Spinal Twists

Practised these lying on your back. Include any other leg exercises.

4. The Forward Bend Pose over both legs

(paschimottanasana)

During pregnancy a similar posture was practised with one leg

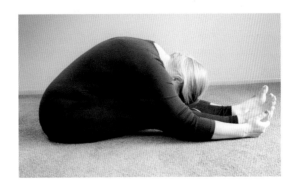

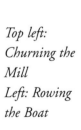

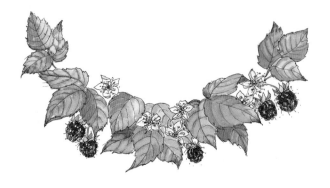

Six Months After the Birth

When your baby is 6 months old, it is safe to include all the exercises and postures recommended for pregnancy. I would also suggest beginning the unmodified form of the Salute to the Sun with the addition of the Cobra which was not included for pregnancy. In addition, I will outline some excellent *asanas* which are appropriate for women at this time as they have particular relevance for balancing the female reproductive system.

1. The Boat
(naukasana)

The Boat is quite a strenuous posture that works deeply into your abdominal muscles. It is very important never to strain, shake, or repeat the exercise so often that you end up with sore abdominal muscles for days after. If you consider that you were pregnant for nine months and now your baby is 6

months old, it is reasonable to presume that these muscles are likely to be a little weak and need to be treated with respect. It is better to gradually increase the number you do over time, so that muscle tone and strength can be developed progressively.

When the Boat is practised correctly, it is fairly demanding. It is important to elevate your legs and body to an equal height. Experiment a little, lifting your legs and body higher or lower, until you eventually find the most balanced and also most demanding position.

You will immediately notice the benefits to your abdominal area, as tone, strength and firmness are improved. The function of your digestive system is enhanced. Regular practise of this posture will bring balance to your nervous system by tensing and relaxing your body. Your back muscles will be strengthened which is particularly important as your

The complete book of
yoga and meditation
for pregnancy

back is often stressed during pregnancy and labour.

1. Lie on your back with your body straight and relaxed.

2. Breathe in as you lift your head, shoulders, arms, feet and legs from the floor, keeping your legs the same height as your head and shoulders. You will resemble a wide 'V', lifting up about 30 cm off the floor.

3. Breathe out as you lower your body to the floor.

4. Repeat this up to five times.

5. Rest and relax when you have completed the practice.

2. The Archer
(dhanurakarshan asana)

The Archer has been included here because of the powerful benefits it gives to your abdominal area, primarily your reproductive system, digestive system, urinary system and bladder. You will notice it stretching and toning your back muscles, hips, spinal column and the hamstring muscles at the back of your legs.

I consider the Archer to be a reasonably strong posture and there will be some people who find it quite difficult. However, it can be modified to suit your own degree of flexibility by using a piece of cloth or a length of flat rope that can be placed around your foot, rather than you trying to reach it. As with any new posture, take a little more time and observe how your body is feeling. At no time force or push yourself beyond what is a natural stretch for the final posture. Loosen and free your hips before you begin by doing the Hip Rotation exercise and the Butterfly.

1. Sit on the floor with your legs stretched out in front of you.

2. Bend your right leg up to near your left thigh, holding onto your right foot or big toe with your right hand.

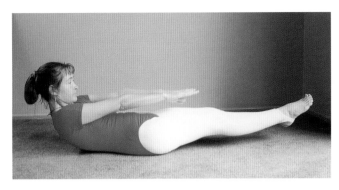

3. Take your left hand down towards your left foot, holding onto your toes if you are able to reach. If you can't reach your foot, make a sling out of a piece of cloth or rope and hold onto that instead.

4. Keeping your elbow above your knee, lift your right foot up

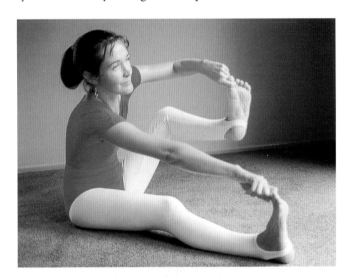

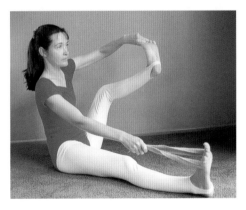

towards your head, bringing your toe as close to your ear as possible. Keep your back as straight as possible in the final posture. Breathe in while lifting your leg up and back towards your ear, breathe out as the posture is relaxed.

5. Repeat this movement up to five times. When your leg is drawn back, it is like the archer's bow expanding and when your leg relaxes it resembles the tension in the bow being released.

6. If you wish to hold the final posture, breathe quietly and remain completely relaxed. Repeat the exercise for the other leg, reversing all the instructions.

3. The Plough Preparation
(poorwa halasana)
Note on the next four positions

The following four postures: the Plough Preparation, the Half Shoulder Stand, the Shoulder Stand and the Plough can be grouped together. Their benefits overlap and they are practised in sequence. I would not usually recommend they be attempted unless under the supervision of a teacher, but if the instructions and precautions are followed carefully there is no reason why they cannot be learnt from a book. It is a matter of taking complete responsibility for what you do and how you are doing it, so that the benefits and rewards can be enjoyed to their fullest.

It is preferable to practise these *asanas* on an empty stomach, or at least three hours after a meal. It is very important to warm your body first before practising any of these new postures. These practices are usually done at the end of the exercise section of a program, when your body is warm, lose and relaxed.

Generally, these postures supply your brain with a rich blood flow, improving concentration and sharpening your memory. While your head is down, blood can drain away from your lower limbs and replenish

your upper body, head and face, while relieving pressure and tiredness from your feet and legs. When the posture is released and the body is returned to the prone position, the lower limbs receive a nourishing supply of blood which results in balance and rejuvenation of your whole being.

The major organs of your digestive system, large intestine and pelvic region, are relieved of pressure, which is useful for conditions such as prolapse, constipation and diverticulitis. Your major organs and your glandular system are revitalised and your nervous system is balanced and strengthened.

When first attempting this group of postures, I would advise only holding the final posture for five breaths at a time and extending that gradually after regular practise.

Caution: These postures are not recommended for people with spinal problems, slipped discs, cardiac and blood pressure disorders. They are excellent postures to do for normalising the health of your thyroid, however, there is a caution for people suffering from thyroid gland dysfunction. If you have a thyroid problem you should not consider doing these exercises unless you have been given the approval of your doctor and are under the care of a teacher who has a reasonable understanding of your medical condition. In the situation of mild thyroid insufficiency I would only recommend the Plough Preparation posture.

The Plough Preparation is a safe and easy preparation for the Plough and the Shoulder Stand. Be very aware of how you are feeling in this posture. If you are experiencing any discomfort don't proceed to the more advanced

208

The complete book of
yoga and meditation
for pregnancy

postures until you feel completely at
ease. If you want more lift in your
pelvis, a small folded blanket or a few
cushions can be placed under your hips
for a greater tilt. For an easier approach,
this posture can be practised with your
buttocks close to a wall and your feet
resting against the wall. When your legs
are in this position they can be tilted
forward to the intended posture before
resting them against the wall when you
need to.

Note: It is important to always
keep your head still in the final postures
and to come out of the postures slowly.

1. Lie on your back with your
buttocks close to a wall. Bend your
knees and place your feet on the wall.
Place your hands in a tight fist under
your buttocks or, for a greater tilt, place
cushions under your buttocks. Your

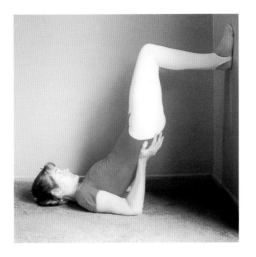

feeling, before
proceeding.

2. When
you are ready, lift
your hips a little
higher and hold
that posture while
you breathe and
relax. This is
really a
supported
Shoulder
Stand.

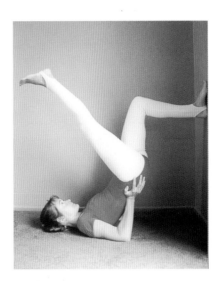

3. If
this posture is comfortable and
there is no feeling of fullness in
your face you can lift your hips
higher to feel your chin pressing
lightly onto your upper chest.
There are many people who find
the Shoulder Stand postures too
uncomfortable, preferring this
supported variation instead. This
will still supply all the benefits of
the more difficult postures but is
much easier to do.

4. With your back flat on
the floor and your hips supported,
ease your legs towards your face,
holding this for a short time before

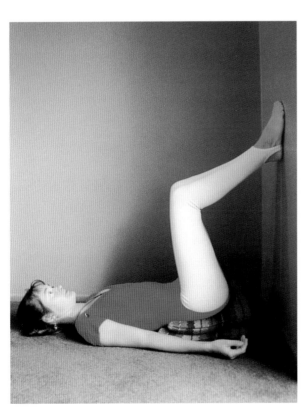

head, shoulders and the middle of your
back remain on the floor throughout
this exercise. Some people like to pause
in this position and adjust to the

returning your legs to the wall. This can
be repeated as often as you like or it can
be held for a short time while breathing
quietly. When your feet are taken away

from the wall, your shoulders and upper body take the full weight of your lower body, which is why it is important to proceed very slowly with the exercise.

5. When you are ready to come out of the posture, remove your hands or cushions from under your hips and roll onto your side to lower your legs to the floor. Rest in a relaxation posture for a few minutes before sitting up or continuing with another posture.

If you notice any discomfort in your lower back after completing this posture, sit with your knees tucked into your chest and your arms wrapped around your legs and gently rock your body from side to side.

4. The Half Shoulder Stand
(vipareeta karani asana)

There are many important benefits to be gained for the whole internal body from practising the Half Shoulder Stand and the Shoulder Stand, primarily because of the inverted position. When the body is inverted or reversed from the usual way of being, the whole internal body is positively effected as pressure is relieved from the internal body and the influence of gravity is therefore greatly reduced. This has many positive effects on all the major systems of the body. For example:

- The digestive system is revitalised and renewed resulting in improved health and better organ function. This means that the stomach and the bowel will operate more efficiently.
- Constipation and haemorrhoids can be relieved with continued practise, while other minor disorders of the small and large intestine will be remedied. This has particular relevance for those suffering with diverticulitis or pockets in the bowel that cause pain, bloating and discomfort in the effected areas. As

the bowel works more efficiently, harmful toxins are removed from the body, resulting in a feeling of increased wellbeing and good health. If there is a predisposition to prolapsed organs, especially in the uterus and the bowel, these postures are an ideal way to prevent the problem becoming worse.

- When the body is in the inverted position, the muscles of the pelvic floor have the weight taken off them. This plays an important role in overcoming any weakness in that part of the body. This is especially true in the event of mild incontinence where regular practice of this posture and the Pelvic Floor exercises will be helpful. The occurrence of urinary tract infections is also reduced with continued practice.
- Sinus congestion, headaches, asthma and other bronchial or upper respiratory tract problems are eased as a healthy blood supply is encouraged to these parts of the body.
- All the inverted postures have a powerful regulating effect on the thyroid and parathyroid glands.
- The muscles of the neck, shoulders and back are encouraged to stay more relaxed. At the same time, an increased blood flow to the chest is beneficial for the function of the heart.
- The endocrine system is balanced, improving overall health and wellbeing.
- If there is a tendency for nervous instability such as anxiety, unreasonable behaviour and uncharacteristic irritability, insomnia and even nervous breakdown, the calming and soothing benefits received from these postures will encourage balanced to be restored

210

The complete book of
yoga and meditation
for pregnancy

quickly and bring relief from these problems.

- I am not suggesting that by simply practising the inverted postures all emotionally related disorders will be alleviated. However, with continued and regular practice of these postures the problems will definitely be reduced over time and balance will be restored to the whole person. Yoga works very deeply and effectively on the internal body and when the endocrine system and the nervous systems are balanced and functioning well, many emotionally related problems can be effectively reduced.

- These excellent postures play a significant role for women as they are specific for restoring and maintaining optimum health in the female reproductive system. They are designed to create tone and strength in the woman's body while superior function is established to the reproductive organs.

In the Half Shoulder Stand your body is held at a 45 degree angle with your eyes in line with your toes. This is the preferred position for beginners. It is important, in the beginning, to be aware of any shortness of breath, restricted breathing or excessive fullness in your face. If any of these symptoms is bothering you, it would be better to discontinue with this practice and spend more time in the Plough Preparation. I don't recommend practising the Shoulder Stand until you feel completely relaxed and safe in the Half Shoulder Stand.

For those suffering from stiffness or tension in the neck, this posture will either work very well to relieve the problem or aggravate the situation. Some people like to place a small piece of foam or thin blanket under the neck for comfort and support.

Note: When the inverted postures are completed, practise a counterpose such as the Fish, the Pelvic Tilt or the Shoulder Pose (detailed below).

1. Begin by lying on your back with your body straight and relaxed. Rest your hands beside your body and breathe regularly.

2. Bend your knees and bring your legs close in to your chest. Place your hands under your hips to support your back. Keep your elbows parallel to your body rather than out to the sides.

3. Lift your hips away from the floor and, keeping your elbows on the floor, balance your hips on your hands so that they are taking the weight of your body. Relax into this position before proceeding. Keep your breathing even and steady.

4. Elevate your legs to a position where your toes are in line with your eyes and your body is 45 degrees off the ground rather than straight up. Keep your hands under your hips. Do not turn your head when you are in the posture or as you come out of it.

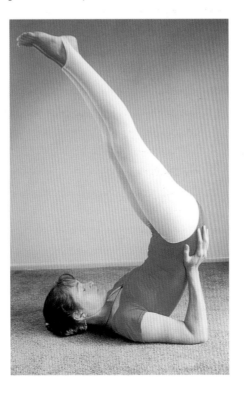

5. Follow procedures 4 to 6 of the Shoulder Stand.

5. The Shoulder Stand
(sarvangasana)

This posture is often known as the 'mother' of all yoga postures. The Sanskrit word *sarvanga* means the whole body, and the practice of *sarvangasana*

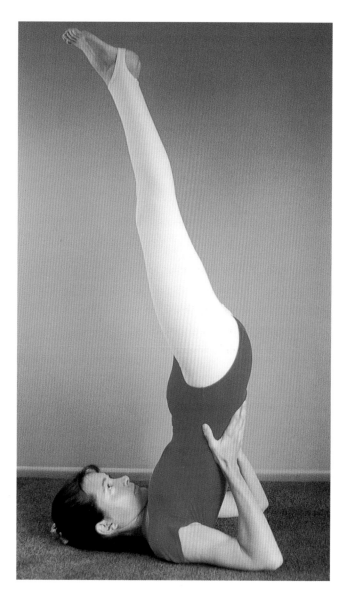

involves your entire body. Approach this posture with care and a sensible attitude, with awareness of how you are feeling during and after the practice.

1. Follow procedures 1 to 3 of the Half Shoulder Stand.

2. When you are ready, straighten your legs and your body so that you are completely erect with your hands firmly supporting the middle of your back. Your body and legs should be in line and your chin pressed against the centre of your chest.

3. Breathe regularly, in a quite and easy manner. Keep your body relaxed, steady and as still as possible. It is very important not to turn your head but to keep it still throughout the whole practice and as you return to the floor.

4. For people who are new to the Shoulder Stands, only hold the posture for one or two minutes or even less if that seems too long. With practise, this time can be extended for as long as you are relaxed and comfortable.

5. Come out of the posture slowly and steadily, taking two breaths to return to the floor. Take a final inhalation in the full posture and, while exhaling, lower your back gently to the floor. Your legs will now be upright and your back flat on the floor. Your hands support your back as it is lowered to the floor. From there, take another inhalation and, as you breathe out, either lower your legs to the floor or bend your legs and bring them into your chest. Your hands can be placed under your buttocks to alleviate back strain and to prevent the middle of your back from arching as your legs are lowered. By coming out of the Shoulder Stand in this way, you have much more control over your movements and reduce the chance of injury.

6. The Shoulder Pose or the Fish can now be practised as a suitable counterpose.

6. The Plough
(halasana)

The Plough is the final inverted posture to be covered in this chapter and it is traditionally practised following the Shoulder Stand. The Sanskrit word *hala* means a plough and when you are in the final posture that is what you will resemble. The middle of your body is contracted so your whole abdominal area is greatly stimulated and massaged. Intestinal gas and bloating are relieved, while any disorders or minor upsets to your digestive system are eliminated. Your spinal column and the muscles of your back and the backs of your legs are stretched.

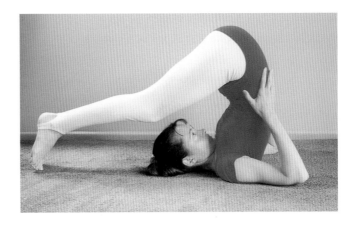

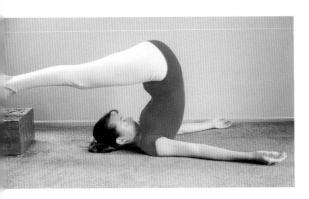

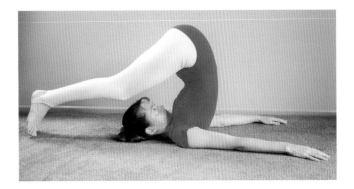

1. Begin in the Half Shoulder Stand or the Shoulder Stand. Keeping your legs straight, lower your legs over your head so that your feet rest on the floor behind your head.

Note: If you are unable to reach the floor with your toes, cushions or a low stool can be placed so that your feet are able to reach as far as possible. Alternatively, place yourself in such a position that your toes come to rest on a couch or a step of the appropriate height. Extend out into the full Plough in your own time.

2. Keep your legs straight and rest your toes on the floor. A reasonable amount of flexibility is required in your back muscles and hamstrings, so remember to only extend as far as your own level of flexibility allows. Your hands can be supporting the middle of your back, extended away from your body along the floor or, if you are confident in the previous two positions, your hands can be placed forward of your body to rest beside your feet.

3. Breathe quietly in the final posture. Relax and be as comfortable as possible. To achieve a more complete Plough, walk your feet away further from your body. This will give a dramatic 'chin lock' and stimulate your thyroid gland.

4. When you want to come out of the posture, support your back with your hands and return to the floor as for the Shoulder Stand.

5. Lie with your knees tucked into your chest and gently massage your back by rocking slowly from side to side. This can be followed by a suitable counterpose such as the Pelvic Tilt, the Fish or the Shoulder Pose.

7. The Fish
(matsyasana)

In Sanskrit the word *matsya* means fish and this posture is dedicated to the fish incarnation of Vishnu, the second deity of the Hindu trilogy. Vishnu's job was to preserve the world and, according to legend, when the world was a very corrupt place and heading for disaster from a universal flood, Vishnu became a fish and warned the leaders and great sages of the impending disaster. This warning saved the world from ruination and the sacred vedic texts from devastation.

The Fish is considered a very important yoga asana and is recommended as an excellent counterpose to all the inverted postures. When the Fish is practised, your body is extended and stretched in the opposite way from the Shoulder Stand and the Plough, balancing your internal body and working the opposing muscle groups. There are a number of variations of the Fish but I will only detail the simpler form. If you find the Fish is not to your liking, or if it causes you discomfort, the Pelvic Tilt, the Shoulder Pose, the Cobra, or the Cat would all be suitable alternatives to do in its place.

Caution: This posture is not suitable for people with neck injuries.

The Fish fully expands your whole chest, relieving respiratory complaints. The front of your body is expanded and stretched. Tense upper back muscles are relaxed and greater flexibility is gained especially in your middle and lower back. With your head held back in the final posture, your thyroid gland is balanced and regulated.

I feel it is worth mentioning that the Fish does not seem to be everybody's favourite posture. There will always be postures that you like more than others but persevering with a posture that is not suitable for you is not the way to go. I am not suggesting you give up on an exercise because you find it

challenging when you first try it, but when there are obvious difficulties and physical limitations simply choose an alternative that better suits your body type and physical history.

1. Lie on your back with your body straight and relaxed. Rest your arms beside you.

2. Arch your back and expand your chest out fully. Leave the crown of your head resting on the floor. Feel the weight of your body evenly balanced between the top of your head, your buttocks and your legs. The expansion of your chest will give a sense of lightness to that part of your body.

3. Hold the final posture for up to five breaths, remaining comfortable and relaxed.

4. Return to the floor by gently lowering your back and shoulders, remembering never to come out of the Fish in a hurry or jerk your neck in any way.

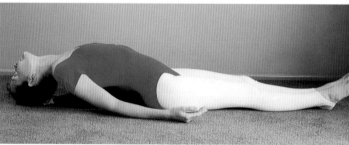

8. The Dynamic Plough
(druta halasana)

This wonderfully invigorating exercise is a combination of two postures, the Seated Forward Bend and the Plough. It is a very powerful exercise to do and as the title suggests it will dynamically tone and stimulate your body and bring greater alertness to your mind. I do not recommend this exercise if you are not reasonably fit, as you might find it exhausting rather than stimulating.

The complete book of
yoga and meditation
for pregnancy

The Dynamic Plough is a complete exercise in itself and the whole body is stretched and toned.

- You will notice all stiffness, tension and fatigue are removed as you become more supple and flexible in your movements.
- The respiration and heart rate are increased with continued practice, making this an extremely beneficial exercise for the cardiovascular system.
- The back and spinal column are well exercised and massaged due to the rolling movement from the tail bone through to the vertebrae in the neck. This has an invigorating effect on the nervous system, enhancing wellbeing and vitality in the whole body.
- The digestive system is toned and balanced, bringing relief to those suffering with intestinal disturbances such as constipation and diarrhoea. It is also highly recommended for people with disorders of the liver, gallbladder, stomach and bowel because it has a regulating and rejuvenating effect on those organs.
- The kidneys and adrenal glands are nourished and restored to health, increasing vitality and energy levels.
- This posture will also improve body tone and remove fat deposits, particularly around the waist and hips.

Variation (i)

1. Sit on the floor with your body straight, your legs in front of you and your arms beside your body.

2. Breathe in and as you breathe out bend forward over your legs into the Forward Stretch. Relax your head towards your legs. Your arms and your shoulders should be loose and your legs straight.

3. Continue to breathe naturally as you return to the seated position, and continue moving as you lift your legs over your head into the Plough. Your hands can be brought in to support your back or they can be extended over your head to meet your feet.

4. From the Plough posture roll your body back again over your legs and into the Forward Bend. Continue to move your body forward and back, repeating this up to nine times. You will build momentum and a flowing movement as your body rolls forward over your legs and back into the Plough.

5. When this is complete, rest with your body in a relaxation posture until your breathing and heartbeat have returned to normal. Some people like to rest with their knees bent after the exercise.

Variation (ii)

1. Begin – as for variation (i) – with your body in a seated position.

2. Breathe in and stretch your arms up above your head. Keep your shoulders relaxed and your spine straight and tall.

3. Breathe out as you extend your body over your legs into the full head to knee position. Stretch your hands towards your feet and rest your head on your legs.

4. Breathe in and return to the upright position, keeping your arms stretched above your head and your spine straight.

5. Breathe out as your legs are taken back into the Plough and your

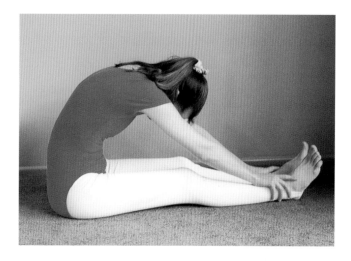

point which makes variation (ii) physically more demanding.

7. To begin with, practise this four or five times and as strength and general fitness levels improve you can increase this number up to nine times or more. As with all yoga exercises, rest when the posture is completed, continuing on with other postures only when your breathing and heart rate have returned to normal.

9. The Sphinx and the Cobra

The Cobra is one of the postures of the Salute to the Sun. I have detailed it in the chapter of that name but I will explain it again here because it is an important *asana* and care needs to be taken when it is practised as a separate posture.

I will also explain the Sphinx posture as this is a halfway posture between the floor and the Cobra, and it can be practised as a preliminary posture before the Cobra. It is also an ideal alternative if there are lower back problems or extreme stiffness in the back.

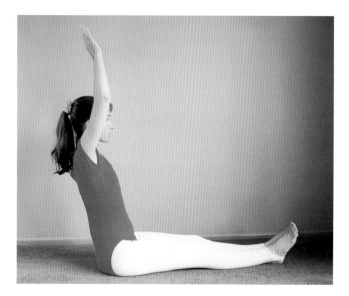

The benefits of the Sphinx and the Cobra are similar. Your back is arched and made more supple, helping to relieve stiffness and inflexibility. Circulation to your spine is improved and your spinal nerves toned. Your kidneys and adrenal glands are toned and enhanced.

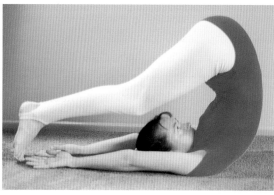

hands are behind your head touching your toes.

6. Continue on in this manner, always straightening your spine and bringing your arms above your head when inhaling. This is the important difference between the two variations and it is this strong lift at the midway

As your back is arched and flexed, the front of your body receives a wonderful stretch, especially through the abdominal and pelvic areas. It is therefore one of the most important *asanas* for the digestive and reproductive systems. The uterus and ovaries are toned, relieving menstrual and gynaecological disorders. Digestion is improved and problems such as mild constipation are alleviated with regular practise, while the bladder is balanced and rejuvenated. The Cobra and, to a lesser degree, the Sphinx are specific postures for women and are especially good six months or so after the birth. They are also extremely valuable before conception for optimum health and wellbeing in these parts of the body.

I feel it is important to remember that you will still benefit from the Cobra whether you are a flexible person by nature, or not. Always practise within your own comfort and flexibility levels. Relax, and enjoy the posture. Once you begin to struggle and force yourself into positions, tension is created in your body making it impossible to breathe into the posture and remain relaxed.

The Sphinx

1. Prepare for the Sphinx by lying on your front with your chin resting on the floor. Rest your lower arms on the floor with your hands flat on the floor beside your face. Keep your legs straight and your feet together.

2. Breathe in as you lift your upper body as high as possible, keeping your lower arms and your hands on the floor. You might need to adjust the position of your hands so that you can remain in this position in complete comfort. Hold the posture and breathe evenly and gently for up to nine breaths. Keep your awareness on your lower back and abdominal area, and relax your body and shoulders.

3. To come out of the Sphinx, breathe in then lower your body to the floor as you breathe out.

The Cobra
(bhujangasana)

Caution: If you have a back problem or are recovering from a recent injury, practise the Sphinx posture rather than the Cobra. It is a much easier position to manage and will not cause discomfort or strain your back.

In the full Cobra posture you will experience a deep stretch throughout the front of your body from the throat to the navel, and a wonderful arch in the whole of your back. Some people

The Sphynx

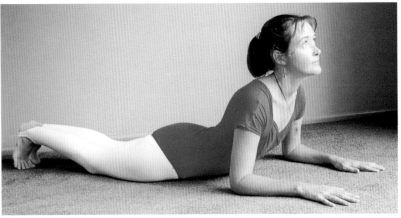

are very flexible in the spine and are able to practise the Cobra effortlessly, whereas others will find they are very stiff in the back and are only able to lift a little higher than the Sphinx.

1. Follow the procedures for the Sphinx. Then, continue to straighten your arms until you have lifted your body as far as you are able without strain or discomfort. It is very important at this point to be completely aware of how you are feeling, never attempting to lift your body higher than you are at ease with. If you find the lift difficult, keep your arms slightly bent in the Cobra and as flexibility increases – with regular practice – you will be able to lift your body a little higher.

2. Lift your body upright. Keep

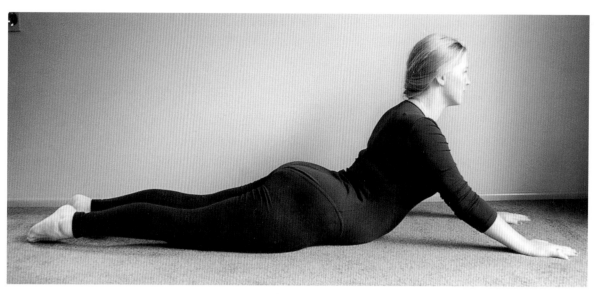

The Cobra

your arms straight, your abdomen and hips on the floor and your shoulders relaxed. If you are completely comfortable in this position and have no neck problems, stretch your head back for the full Cobra. Remain relaxed, breathing quietly for up to nine breaths, or as long as you are comfortable. When you first practise the Cobra you might prefer to hold it for two or three breaths then extend the hold as you become more flexible.

3. Lower your body to the floor as you breathe out.

4. Rest in the Pose of the Child, breathing gently.

10. The Bow
(dhanurasana)

The Sanskrit word *dhanu* means a bow. In this posture your hands pull on your legs, resembling a bow string being pulled back to release an arrow. The Bow works in a similar way to the Cobra, where your back is strongly arched and your abdominal area is toned and stretched. The action of your hands on your feet causes your thigh muscles, your abdominal area, and your whole chest and upper back to be

worked deeply, while your spinal column is made flexible and strong. It is an important posture for women of all ages, as the organs of your reproductive system are internally massaged and toned, thereby restoring regular function.

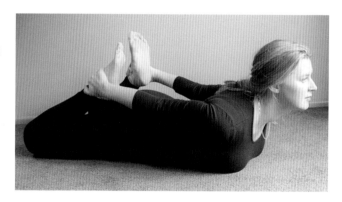

Some people find lifting their legs and upper body at the same time quite hard to do. If this is the case, lift your upper body separately from your lower body until you can feel the lift is done easily and in a relaxed manner. It is important to stay relaxed when practising the Bow. Sometimes I feel people try too hard, tensing the body in an attempt to obtain the lift, instead of staying relaxed and 'light'. Remember to approach it slowly and without struggle, and all difficulties will soon be forgotten.

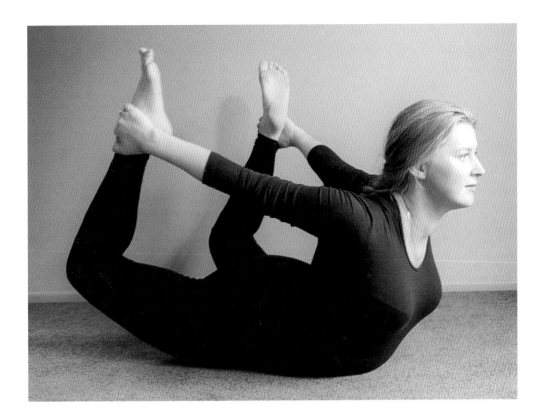

1. Lie on your front with your legs a little apart, your knees bent and your hands holding onto your feet. If you are quite flexible in your back and are wanting a bigger lift, hold onto your ankles instead of your feet.

2. Inhale as you lift your legs, chest and head from the floor. Lift your legs and upper body as high as possible. Your pelvic and abdominal areas are the only part of your body remaining on the floor.

3. Exhale as your body is lowered to the floor. After resting, repeat this up to five times. If you find the Bow easy to do, hold the posture while breathing calmly and regularly.

4. When you have completed the Bow, relax in the Pose of the Child.

11. The Shoulder Pose (kandharasana)

The Shoulder Pose is very similar in application to the Pelvic Tilt which I recommended for pregnancy, the only difference being that the arch in your back is quite a lot higher for this posture. As it has a more dramatic

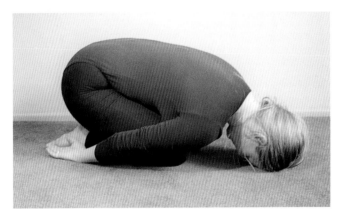

impact on your body than the Pelvic Tilt, it is not recommended for people with abdominal disorders such as peptic ulcers or hernias.

The Shoulder Pose has many benefits for your respiratory, digestive and reproductive systems, while it is also a therapeutic practise for your back and the health of your spinal column.

For people suffering from all upper respiratory tract disorders, asthma or bronchitis, this is an excellent posture to practice on a regular basis. As with all postures that lock your chin into your chest – such as the Plough and the Shoulder Stand – this exercise will be

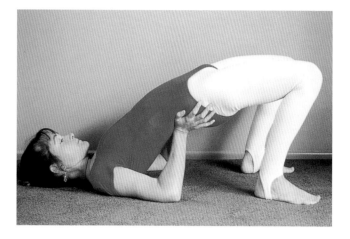

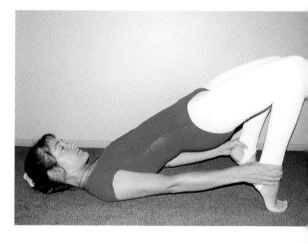

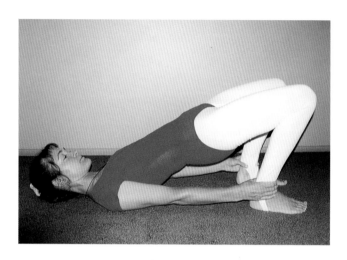

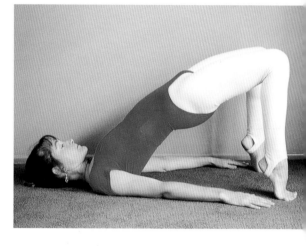

useful for thyroid dysfunction. Any minor disturbances in your digestive system are corrected and regular function retored, especially in the colon, stomach and other major organs of that system, due to the position of the body and the full stretch felt in the abdominal area. Regular practice will assist in overcoming such problems as constipation, indigestion and flatulance. The health of your reproductive system is greatly improved, while the Shoulder Pose is an ideal practice for women who are wanting to conceive but have had a previous history of miscarriage. The muscles of your back, your spinal column and spinal nerves are all benefited and this posturte is highly recommended for people with constant backache and tight shoulders.

1. Lie on your back with your knees bent, your feet hip-distance apart and as close to your buttocks as possible. Rest your arms beside your body and breathe naturally.

2. Lift your hips as high as possible and feel your chin 'locked' close into your chest. Your hands can be placed under your hips to increase the height of the lift or you can hold onto your ankles if you can reach them. The length of your arms will determine whether you reach your ankles or not. It is something that is related to your anatomy rather than degree of flexibility. If you are unable to reach, a piece of wide rope or a strip of material can be wrapped around your ankles to make up the difference in arm length. In either of these positions your heels can be lifted off the ground to accentuate the lift.

The complete book of
yoga and meditation
for pregnancy
∽

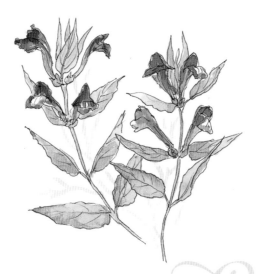

Salute to the Sun
(surya namskara)

Salute to the Sun is an excellent way to warm and loosen your body before practising other yoga exercises. It is comprised of 12 separate yoga *asana*s (postures) gracefully integrated so that one movement follows the other. Breathing, physical exercise, concentration and awareness are beautifully combined into a moving expression of yoga. When your body is stretching in one direction, it is simultaneously flexing in the other. The breathing unifies the movements, breathing in for one posture and breathing out for the next, where the chest expands and contracts rhythmically in time with the movements. This results in a greatly increased uptake and utilisation of oxygen and *prana* within the body and mind.

I suggest you begin quite slowly so as to familiarise yourself with the way the postures flow and to synchronise your breathing with the movements. Practising slowly will enable you to be more aware of the deep stretch in some of the postures. If it is some time since you have done any physical exercise, you might feel lightheaded or breathless when first attempting Salute to the Sun. Although not a frequent occurrence, dizziness or slight nausea can also be experienced. By practising slowly and regularly, this discomfort will go away as your level of fitness gradually increases.

It is up to you how many times you practise this exercise and how quickly or slowly it is completed. Some people prefer to proceed fairly slowly, practising it four or five times. Others choose to do it quite fast, ten times or more. The physical benefits are greater to the cardiovascular system when the sequence is practised quickly but the stretch is deeper and more complete if extra time is taken in each position. I have found the most benefits are gained when this exercise is practised three or four times slowly, taking two or three breaths in each position, then three or four times more quickly, incorporating the correct breathing into each movement.

Generally, this exercise can be safely practised by women of all ages and fitness levels, with obvious consideration to the specific needs of the individual. Always remember to be aware of how you are feeling. Rest if you start to feel uncomfortable, then continue at a comfortable pace until your body adjusts to the exercise.

One full round of Salute to the Sun consists of completing the 12 movements, twice. The first time your right leg is taken back in the Equestrian posture. The second time, take your left leg back. Although this might differ slightly from other teachings, I have found it the easiest way to remember which leg to take back, and to keep track of how many rounds have been done.

When you have completed the desired number of rounds, always lie on the floor in a relaxation position or the Corpse posture, resting until your heart rate and breathing have stabilised and returned to normal.

Benefits
- The heart rate is increased providing quite an aerobic effect. The more Salute to the Sun is performed, the greater the aerobic effect. It is considered a dynamic yoga exercise, where care needs to be taken not to overextend yourself. It is of the utmost importance to always proceed at your own pace.
- As respiration is improved due to deeper and more efficient breathing, all the cells of the body are replenished and revitalised with a healthy blood supply and *prana*

(energy). The breathing becomes more efficient as you will naturally be inclined to inhale and exhale to a greater capacity and depth. This increases the uptake of oxygen as you inhale and helps remove carbon dioxide as you exhale. When breathing improves, the lungs can more easily displace and remove any stale air that often remains at the base of the lungs.

- Circulation to all parts of the body is increased. The brain receives a fresh supply of oxygenated blood, bringing freshness to the mind and clarity to the thoughts. Cerebral circulation is improved when your head is down, helping to improve the memory, increase alertness and awareness.
- A more enriched blood supply to the major organs of the digestive system is provided, resulting in improved organ function and efficiency. Conditions such as a sluggish digestion, constipation, indigestion and many other imbalances of the digestive system can be rectified. Function to all the major organs is improved, especially the liver, spleen, pancreas, kidneys, heart and lungs.
- When respiratory and circulatory systems are working better, the skin receives a greater blood flow. As the skin is one of the major channels of elimination for the body toxins are more efficiently removed and the skin will glow with health and vitality.
- During the practice of Salute to the Sun, the abdominal organs are alternately stretched and compressed, helping to ensure optimum organ function.
- Congestion is removed from the whole body.
- The endocrine system is stimulated and balanced.

222

The complete book of
yoga and meditation
for pregnancy

- All muscle groups are exercised and toned, bringing relief to stiff muscles. Muscle tension is quickly removed.
- Excess fat is removed as the body is toned and made firm.
- The spine, central nerves and back muscles are toned and strengthened. With regular practise, the spine

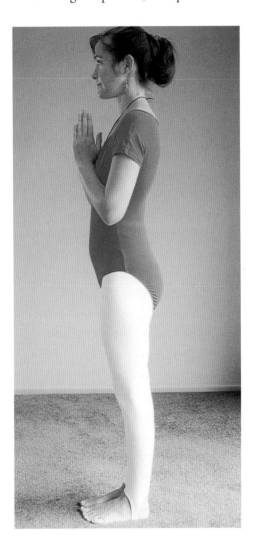

becomes more supple and flexible which is so important to the health and fitness of the whole body.

- The hamstring tendons and calf muscles are stretched and circulation to the feet and legs is greatly improved.
- With regular practice of this exercise, mental and physical fatigue are relieved and a much greater sense of balance will be felt throughout the whole body, mind and spirit.

1. The Prayer
(pranamasana)

Stand with your feet together and your body straight. Join the palms of your hands at the centre of your chest. Relax and breathe quietly. Before you begin, take three deep yoga breaths to become centred and focused.

2. Raised Arms
(hasta uttanasana)

Breathe in while raising your arms above your head, arching your body slightly back from the standing position. Stretch deeply throughout your abdominal area, extending through your arms to your finger tips. If you have a very stiff back or are experiencing back problems, stand with your feet further apart and do not extend back as far.

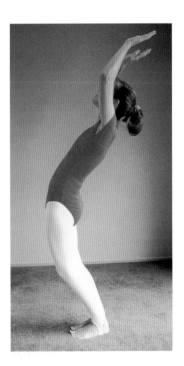

3. Forward Bend
(padahastasana)

Breathe out and bend your body forward. Stretch your hands towards your feet, and the top of your head is facing the floor. Hold your legs straight but not tight, and have your shoulders and neck relaxed. The weight of your head will gently stretch the muscles of your neck so it is important to be aware of the position of your head, allowing it to hang freely between your arms. If you are unable to reach the floor with your hands, do not strain or overextend your body, as this can result in damage to

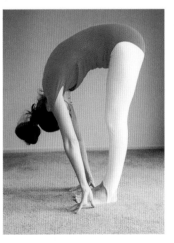

your hamstrings and back. It is more important to be aware that you are relaxed, and your body is stretching to its natural capacity.

4. The Equestrian
(ashwa sanchalanasana)

Breathe in and take your right leg back so that the toes of your right foot and your right knee are on the floor.

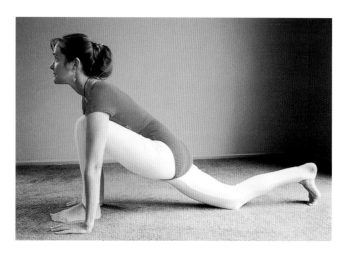

The left leg is bent and your foot is flat on the floor. Place your hands on the floor either side your left foot. In this posture the lunge is deep into your hip as you lean forward over your left leg, while a full extension is felt throughout your right hip and leg.

5. The Mountain
(parvatasana)

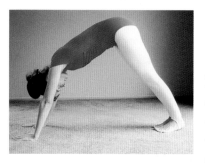

Exhale as you take your left leg back to your right foot. Your feet can be together or slightly apart with your heels as close to the floor as possible. Relax your head and neck between your shoulders, and draw your hips back away from your hands, thereby obtaining a deep stretch throughout your legs, back and arms. As greater flexibility is achieved, your heels will come closer to the floor without

changing the position of your feet or your hands.

6. The Salute with 8 Limbs
(ashtanganamaskra)

As you breathe out, lower your body to the floor. Touch the floor with your toes, knees, chest, chin and hands. This position gets its name because eight parts of your body are touching

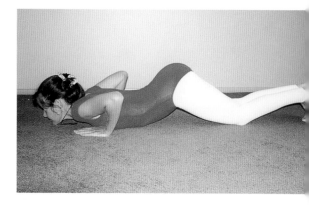

the floor. The pelvis, hips and abdominal area should not be in contact with the floor. This movement is the way to progress from position 6 to position 7.

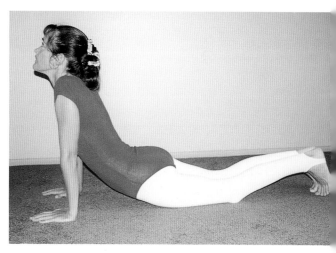

7. The Cobra
(bhujangasana)

Breathe in as you straighten your arms and lift your body from the floor. This will form an arch in your back. Be aware not to arch your back further than is comfortable as this will only cause tension. For some people who are

224

The complete book of
yoga and meditation
for pregnancy

not very loose or flexible in the back, your arms will remain slightly bent in the final position. With time and practise your back will gradually loosen so that your arms can be straightened. Your hips and pelvis remain in contact with the floor, and your head is only taken back if you have the flexibility to do so and if you are free from injury or tension in your neck.

8. The Mountain
(parvatasana)

Breathe out and return to the Mountain Pose, position 5.

9. The Equestrian
(ashwa sanchalanasana)

Breathe in and return to position 4, stepping your left foot in between your hands as your right leg is extended back.

10. Forward Bend
(padahastasana)

Breathe out as you step both feet together. Keep your head down with your neck, shoulders and arms relaxed. Your legs remain straight in the forward bend, as in position 3.

11. Raised Arms
(hasta uttanasana)

Breathe in as your body is raised to the upright standing position, taking your arms above your head, arching back slightly to repeat position 2.

If you have a weak or injured back, I recommended bending your knees slightly as your body is returned to the standing position when moving from position 10 to 11. This will help prevent extra strain on your back muscles, while it greatly reduces the extent of the stretch in your hamstrings.

12. The Prayer
(pranamasana)

Breathe out for the final posture, bringing the palms of your hands together in centre of your chest for the Prayer position. Your body should be straight and relaxed.

This completes half of one round of Salute to the Sun. Continue on, following all the details, remembering to take your left leg back in positions 4 and 9 for the second side. This will give equal stretch to both sides of your body and completes one round of Salute to the Sun.

When you have completed the number of rounds you wish to do, always rest on the floor in the relaxation position, until your breathing and heart rate have returned to normal. When you feel quiet and relaxed take a few slow, deep yoga breaths and visualise *prana* (energy) moving through your body, mind and spirit. This completes the postnatal exercise program. I hope you continue to enjoy your yoga practices, and find a place for yoga on life's busy path. I am sure you will have a lifetime filled with precious moments and wonderful adventures as you and your child share this memorable journey together as mother and child.

This completes the postnatal exercise program. I hope you continue to enjoy your yoga practices, and find a place for yoga on life's busy path. I am sure you will have a lifetime filled with precious moments and wonderful adventures as you and your child share this memorable journey together as mother and child.

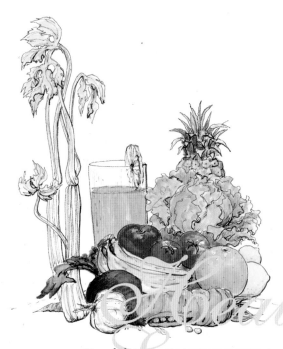

Healthy Eating

The importance of a healthy diet before conception, during pregnancy and after birth cannot be emphasised enough. The type and quality of foods eaten during these times have an unquestionable influence on a woman's health, her baby's health *in utero* and after the birth.

Ideally, the concept of a well-balanced diet is something that both parents would be wise to consider before they plan to conceive. The health of both the mother and the father has an important bearing on the health of the child. In many ways, optimum nutrition by both parents prior to conception is as important as the mother's health during pregnancy, if not more so because the foundations of a healthy child are laid in those months preceding conception.

When a couple are planning a pregnancy, they have the opportunity to make the necessary adjustments to their

diet and to ensure it is as healthy and nutritious as possible. The emphasis needs to be on eating natural, healthy, simple foods that are still very tasty and acceptable to the individual palate. Your local doctor, chemist and health food store would have up to date information on a well-balanced diet and on which foods to avoid.

Unless you are nutritionally deficient or under extreme stress, most of your daily nutritional requirements can be met by food rather than nutritional supplements. We are all different and therefore our nutritional requirements can vary considerably. Be sure that your diet is nutritionally balanced for your own individual needs.

Eating a well-balanced diet involves taking extra care about what you are eating and being discerning about the quality of the foods you buy. To successfully meet the necessary daily requirements, buy fresh fruit and vegetables that are free from chemicals

226

The complete book of
yoga and meditation
for pregnancy

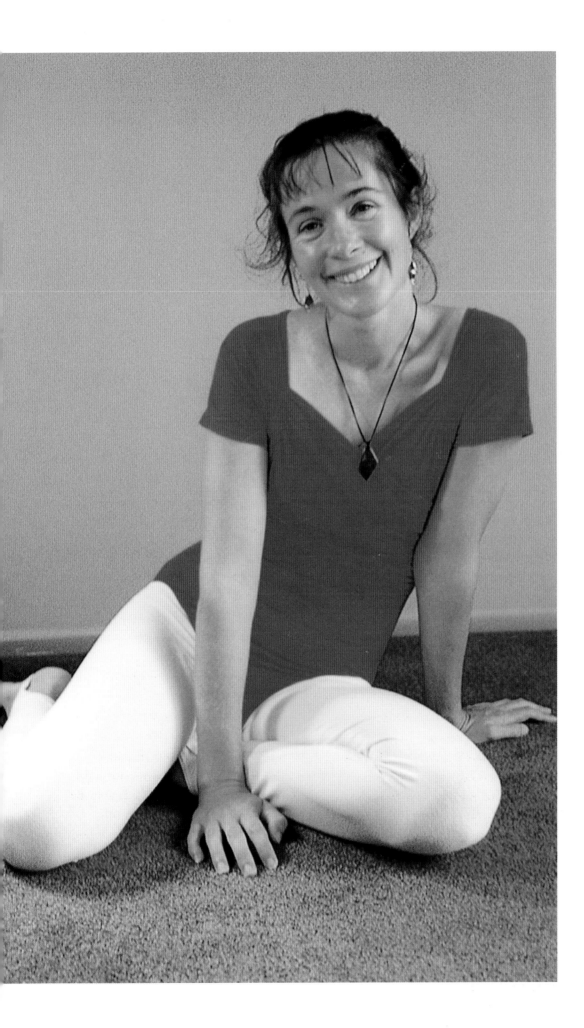

Healthy eating

and sprays if possible. Include juices and other dynamic foods in your daily diet, especially if you are on a vegetarian or vegan diet.

The information detailed is only a general outline and not an in-depth study. For more information on these topics, refer to the books recommended in the Bibliography or speak to a qualified Naturopath or Nutritionist.

Fresh fruit and vegetables

Eat two or three pieces of fresh, in-season fruit each day. Choose fresh seasonal vegetables and eat them either lightly steamed or baked. Eat plenty of fresh raw salads.

Other than the traditional salad vegetables such as lettuce, cucumber and tomato, there are plenty of vegetable that can be eaten raw or made into salads. Try finely grated zucchini, beetroots, carrots, spinach, red and green peppers and other leafy green vegetables. When carrots and beetroots are grated raw it's amazing how sweet and juicy they are. Even small pieces of cauliflower and broccoli can be added to your salads. The variety of salad combinations is unlimited, providing you with the opportunity to create interesting and nutritious salads which can be topped off with tasty dressings.

Some people find it difficult to digest raw foods when they are first introduced to the diet, so it is best to increase the quantities of raw food gradually to avoid digestive problems. There are a number of excellent books available that explain the ways to prepare tasty and wholesome meals using raw foods.

Juices

Fresh fruits and vegetables can be made into juices which are a wonderful source of vital enzymes, vitamins and minerals in a concentrated, easily digestible form. When making juices, always dilute the amount of juice with water by at least half, particularly beetroot and carrot juice. Undiluted they can sometimes cause slight nausea and discomfort because their high sugar concentrations place an extra load on the liver and the pancreas. This is easy to understand when you think that under normal circumstances you might eat only half a carrot or a few slices of beetroot at one time. Always remember to sip the juice slowly as it is a concentrated food source that needs to be introduced into the body gradually. Also, place a piece of ice in the glass before the juice to prevent oxidation.

I prefer not to combine vegetable and fruit juices in the same drink because the fruits take less time to digest and will therefore leave the stomach sooner than the vegetables. When they are drunk in combination, gas can sometimes cause uncomfortable bloating.

There have been many important and valuable books written on the curative value of juices. The juices I have found to be the most beneficial for pregnant women and nursing mothers are the following:

Beetroot juice helps to build up the red blood cells and is therefore very useful if your iron levels are low or if you have a history of anaemia. The leaves are said to be very useful for women in general, being high in iron. Beetroot juice is very good for the liver, gall bladder and

228

The complete book of
yoga and meditation
for pregnancy

kidneys. It is best taken in small amounts, diluted 50 percent with water. Choose small beetroots rather than the larger ones which are inclined to be bitter.

Carrot juice is probably the most well known and popular of all juices and is often used by itself, or mixed with other juices. It is very high in vitamin A and is valuable for the whole digestive system, as a cleanser and purifier for the skin and blood and for healthy eyes.

Carrot juice is a tonic for improving breast milk quantity and quality. As a general guideline I would add two small beetroots – including the greens if they look alive and healthy – to three or four good sized carrots. Then dilute the juice by half with water.

Celery juice is a cleanser for the whole body. It neutralises acids and restores the sodium/potassium levels in the body. It is also very high in organic sodium, calcium and a host of other minerals. The cooling property of celery makes it especially useful if the last months of your pregnancy are during the summer and you feel you are 'overheating'. Adding celery juice to your daily juices could be very helpful if you suffer from edema and swelling of the feet and ankles in hot weather. Celery juice combines well with beetroot and carrot over crushed ice.

Cucumber is another 'cooling' vegetable that is also a natural diuretic. This last point is worth considering if you have puffy fingers and swollen feet in the last trimester. Cucumber is high in the mineral potassium which is involved in keeping the fluid levels in the body stable and balanced. It is also recommended if you have high blood pressure.

English spinach makes a wonderful juice either by itself or – better still – added to any of the other vegetable juices mentioned. It is a valuable cleanser and acts to restore balance to the whole digestive system. Spinach has generous amounts of vitamin A, B6, E, and K, it is extremely high in iron and folic acid and has substantial amounts of zinc and calcium.

Taking spinach in this way means you are digesting much larger quantities than if you were to have, for example, a spinach salad or steamed spinach. This is so beneficial if you are needing to increase your iron levels and wish to do that through your food rather than with supplements. It contains generous amounts of Folic acid, which is extremely important for women over 30, as it plays a vital role in reducing the incidence of spina bifida in babies.

Fruit juices made from lemon, grapefruit, orange, apple, pear, mango, watermelon and pineapple make a healthy and nutritious alternative to that afternoon cup of tea or coffee.

Garlic and onions

Include garlic and onions in your cooking every day as they are medicines in themselves. Garlic and the whole onion family contain abundant amounts of the mineral sulphur which acts as a cleanser and antiseptic to the digestive system. Garlic is well known as an effective detoxifier and blood purifying agent, while it is also a very powerful digestive aid. However, in breastfed infants garlic and onions sometimes cause colic in the first three months so if you are breast feeding and your baby has colic it might be worth removing these foods from your diet until your baby is a little older.

Lean meat, chicken, fish and eggs

Include in your diet lean meats such as chicken (minus the skin and free range if possible) trimmed lamb and beef if you eat red meat, and fresh deep sea fish at least twice a week. This will provide you with protein and other necessary nutritional requirements. Always attempt to find out where the fish was caught, and if possible select fish from waters that are as unpolluted as possible. Fish is low in calories and very high in protein and is much easier for the body to digest than red meats and chicken.

Although I do not like recommending tinned foods, when tinned salmon, tuna and sardines are included to your diet, they provide exceptionally rich sources of calcium and phosphorous, especially when the bones are eaten as well.

When choosing eggs try to obtain fresh free-range eggs. They will cost a little more but are better for you. The chickens who laid these eggs are happier and live in a more natural environment, scratching about in the dirt for worms and other tasty treats that especially appeal to chickens. Battery hens, on the other hand, never feel the earth beneath their feet or know the difference between day or night. If you have the space and the time to have your own chickens, they will provide you with a fairly continuous supply of this excellent food source and it's also a sensible way to recycle your own food scraps. Chickens, also, make wonderful pets!

Sprouts

Sprouted grains and legumes will provide your body with predigested protein and a high level of vitamins and minerals. They are a perfectly balanced food within themselves, containing minerals and vitamins that are easy for your body to digest and assimilate. They are an energy-packed live food in an easy to use form. They can be included in your salads and sandwiches or you can sprinkle them on soups and stews. However, like garlic and onions, if your baby has colic when breastfeeding, it might be the sprouts that are causing the problem.

Include alfalfa, mung beans, aduki beans, fenugreek, radish and lentils. All of these make delicious sprouts. Sometimes soya beans and chick peas can also be successfully sprouted under the right conditions. It is common to see many of these sprouts in the supermarkets today, or better still, buy the dry ingredients and sprout your own.

Always eat the fresh sprouts as soon as they begin to show their little green shoots. You can eat them for the next three or four days after which time the nutritional value begins to diminish.

Nuts

Nuts and seeds are another important food group as they provide a rich supply of stored vitality and energy in an easy to obtain and delicious form. They are abundant in concentrated proteins, vitamins and minerals. They are high in the minerals phosphorous and magnesium which are important for the health of your nervous system, as well as calcium, iron, vitamins A, E and the B vitamins. Although they are high in fats, they are especially good for those on vegetarian and vegan diets who might find it more difficult to obtain adequate protein from their diets. They are also useful for people trying to gain weight due to their high calorie levels.

When buying nuts be sure to buy fresh products and if possible eat them directly from their shells. Always chew

230

The complete book of
yoga and meditation
for pregnancy

them thoroughly as this will assist with the digestion process. Pecans, almonds, walnuts and brazil nuts are all easy to obtain. Pine nuts have the highest available protein of all the nuts and are delicious when eaten as a snack or added to salads, rice dishes and vegetable casseroles. If you really enjoy eating nuts, this particular group are also lower in calories than cashew nuts and peanuts.

If you are a peanut butter fiend like me, always buy it freshly made from a health food store so there is a better chance that the peanuts were not rancid when the peanut butter was manufactured. Avoid the commercial products as they have emulsifiers, flavours, hydrogenated oils and preservatives added which are extremely bad for your arteries and heart.

If you are a real peanut butter enthusiast try making your own and if you still need the salty taste add vegetable salt rather than regular salt. All the other nuts mentioned here can be made into tasty nut butters too.

There are many different types of seeds that can be added to savoury and sweet recipes, to improve the taste and aroma but which will also assist the body with the digestion of our foods. These include aniseed, caraway, cardamom, coriander, cumin, dill, fennel, mustard, poppy and pepper to name a few of the most popular and more commonly used.

Sesame seeds, pumpkin seeds and sunflower seeds are in the same class as nuts for supplying vitamins, minerals and protein. Like nuts they are rich in phosphorous, iron and magnesium, which are essential minerals for the bones, teeth, nervous system and the blood vessels. They also contain high levels of the mineral zinc which is so

important for the health of the whole reproductive system in both women and men. It is an important mineral for the health of the immune system, particularly during times of stress.

Sesame seeds are a highly alkaline food and a protein source that is much easier to digest and assimilate than the protein found in meats. Sesame seeds are also made into tahini, a seed butter or paste used in middle eastern cuisine. Tahini can be eaten as a replacement for butter on bread or crackers, especially if you are allergic to dairy products or are looking for something more nutritious to put on your bread. When tahini is added to cooked chick peas, lemon juice and garlic it makes the very tasty and highly nutritious food called humus.

In Turkey the sesame seed is favoured by the men as a general tonic and for added energy and vitality, while in African countries it provides a very important source of protein. I like to add tahini to my salad dressings as it gives a rich, creamy texture and an interesting nutty flavour. It also makes a nutritious alternative milk drink, by adding a teaspoon of tahini to purified water and mixing until completely blended.

Pumpkin seeds and sunflower seeds are rich in the same nutrients as sesame seeds and also very high in the mineral silicon. Both make excellent nut milks and you will find details of the recipe at the end of this chapter.

Grains

Grains such as brown rice, millet, buckwheat, rye, wheat and other whole grain cereals are important sources of fuel for your body. When buying wheat and rye, buy stone ground products because the steel rollers usually involved in the milling process destroy much of the vitamin content contained in the grain. Buy breads containing the whole grain which includes the fibrous outer husks and the valuable wheatgerm. Although these breads are usually more expensive, if you are going to eat bread it is better for your health to obtain whole grain whenever possible.

Rolled oats in the form of muesli or porridge will give you a rich source of the mineral chromium which is involved in energy and glucose metabolism and the regulation of blood sugar.

If you are inclined to miss meals or eat refined foods that are high in sugars, your blood sugar levels will rise and fall dramatically resulting in all the unpleasant symptoms of hypoglycemia or low blood sugar. By starting the day with a hearty bowl of porridge and a little honey you will have all the energy you require for the whole morning and prevent any of the symptoms associated with low blood sugar. Oats are very high in iron and calcium and are also a rich source of the B vitamins.

Another grain to include is millet which is still a popular food in northern European countries and in Asia. I discovered millet when I was pregnant with my first son Ezra and found it to be a pleasant change from porridge. Millet is high in protein and a good energy food and it seems a little lighter to eat than porridge, especially in the summer months.

Dairy products

There are often health problems and allergies associated with consuming dairy products and especially an excess of them. Many people have mild reactions that they are quite unaware of until they eliminate dairy products from their diets and notice a marked improvement in their general health.

There are appetising alternatives to drinking cow's milk and a number of other ways to obtain calcium from your diet. Soya milk, nut milks or goat's milk make acceptable alternatives. Yoghurt, cottage cheese and whey are better for you and easier to digest than milk, cream and cheese and have all the protein, calcium, phosphorous and other vitamins and minerals that are beneficial to our health. When choosing a yoghurt, check that it has the acidophilus strains of 'good' bacteria which assist in keeping the bowel healthy.

Water

Water is essential for maintaining good health and to help flush your body. Drink clean fresh water regularly throughout the day. There are now many water purifiers on the market which remove much of the chemical and biological health hazards. Even if you are travelling overseas, clean bottled water is readily available, an important fact to consider especially when travelling in heavily populated countries.

Soya products

The soya bean is probably one of the best sources of protein available. It can be used in a number of different ways to provide interesting and healthy eating. Soya products can be eaten in the form of tofu and tempeh, in casseroles, in stir fry with other vegetables, in the form of a thick paste called miso, as soya milk, soya flour, soya oil and also soya sprouts. Although they are not as easy to sprout as other grains and legumes, they are worth the effort and patience involved. Their mineral content is more than adequate and they are high in calcium, iron and phosphorous, and they also help to

232

The complete book of
yoga and meditation
for pregnancy

control fats and cholesterol in your body.

Tofu is available in most supermarkets and health food shops and although it is rather bland on its own it is an interesting and very nutritious food when prepared with a bit of imagination.

If you have travelled to Indonesia you might have discovered the unique taste of tempeh which is made from mixing cooked soya beans with an edible fungus, resulting in a compact loaf. In this form, the soya bean is much easier to digest and has an unusual taste that some people think is similar to chicken. Like tofu, it is better prepared before cooking to enhance the taste, by marinating first in mirin and tamari. (Mirin is made from sweet brown rice, water, rice, koji and sea salt. Tamari is a naturally fermented, traditionally made soya sauce which has a much reduced salt content). When soya is made into tempeh, the vitamin B12 content is increased, which is an important consideration for vegetarians and vegans.

It is better to either eat the soya beans as sprouts, tofu and tempeh as they can cause digestive problems when simply boiled. If you decide to use them in casseroles, firstly soak the dried beans overnight and then boil in fresh water before adding the cooked beans to other recipes.

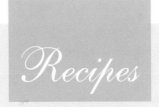

Recipes

Healthy Nut Milk

The nut milk is a delicious and highly nutritious protein drink. It is especially useful during busy times or when you are not be so hungry but know you need to maintain good nutrition. Nut milk is of particular value when breastfeeding, as it will assist with the volume of milk produced and also to create high quality breast milk.

Almonds, pecans, sunflower seeds, pumpkin seeds and cashews are good for making nut milk.

Soak half a cup of nuts and seeds in filtered water or in pure fruit juice, over night. In the morning, blend them with enough water or juice to make a smooth creamy drink. Add to this, one or two teaspoons of brewer's yeast and a little tahini.

This recipe will make enough for two days. Store in the refrigerator in an air tight container.

Creamy Salad Dressing

In a jar, mix one cup of cold pressed olive oil, the juice of one or two lemons, three cloves of fresh garlic finely chopped or crushed, two teaspoons of tahini, a little apple cider vinegar, freshly ground black pepper, vegetable salt and a little brown sugar or honey. Adjust the amounts to suit your tastes. Shake the jar vigorously before each serve and keep in the refrigerator.

BIBLIOGRAPHY

Airola, Paavo 1979, *Every Woman's Book, Health Plus.*

Balaskas, Janet 1989, *New Active Birth*, Thorsons Publishing Group, London.

Bolen, Jean Shinoda 1994, *Crossing to Avalon: A Woman's Midlife Pilgrimage*, Harper Collins, San Fransisco.

Charmine, Susan E. (Ed.) 1989 *The Complete Book of Juice Therapy*, Thorsons Publishing Group, London.

Choedzong, Sakya Losal 1996, Samatha Meditation, *Tibetan Buddhist Society of Canberra*, Canberra.

Chopra, Deepak 1993, *Creating Affluence, New World Library*, California.

Chopra, Deepak 1990, *Perfect Health, Bantam Books*, London.

Dalai Lama 1994, *The Way to Freedom*, Harper Collins, New York.

Dyer, Wayne 1997, *Manifest Your Destiny*, Harper Collins, New York.

Fontana, David 1993, *The Secret Language of Symbols*, Pavilion Books, London.

Hall, Dorothy 1976, *The Natural Health Book*, Nelson, Melbourne.

Hall, Dorothy 1980, *The Dorothy Hall Herb Tea Book*, The Pythagorean Press, Sydney.

Hutchinson, Ronald 1974, *Yoga: A Way of Life*, Hamlyn, Middlesex.

Iyengar, B. K. S. 1966, *Light on Yoga*, George Allen & Unwin, London.

Jensen, Bernard, 1978, *Nature Has a Remedy*, Bernard Jensen, USA.

Kenton, L. & S. 1986, *Raw Energy*, Doubleday, Sydney.

Khyentse, Dilgo 1994, *The Wish Fulfilling Jewel*, Shambhala, Boston.

Kloss, Jethro 1946 *Back to Eden*, Back to Eden Books, California.

Krystal, Phyllis 1989, *Cutting the Ties that Bind*, Element Books, Longmead, Great Britain.

Last, Walter 1977, *Heal Yourself*, Health Print, New Zealand.

Naish, F. & Roberts J. 1996, *The Natural Way to Better Babies*, Random House, Sydney.

Selected Words of His Holiness the Dalai Lama, 1992, Margaret Gee, Sydney.

Sellman, Per & Gita 1981, *The Complete Sprouting Book*, Turnstones Press Limited, Northamptonshire.

Shri Yogendra 1977, *Hatha Yoga Simplified*, The Yoga Institute, Bombay, India.

Sogyal Rinpoche 1994a, *Meditation*, Rider Books, London.

Sogyal Rinpoche 1994b, *The Tibetan Book of Living and Dying*, Rider Books, London.

Swami Satyananda in, Yoga Nidra, Deep Relaxation, 1978, Satyananda Ashrams Australia, Gosford NSW.

Vogel, H. C. A. 1990, *The Nature Doctor*, Mainstream, Edinburgh.

Walker, Barbara 1995, *The Women's Dictionary of Symbols and Sacred Objects*, Pandora, USA.

Walker, Barbara 1983, *The Women's Encyclopedia of Myths and Secrets*, Harper Collins, New York.

Wimala, Bhante Y. 1998, *Lessons of the Lotus*, Judy Paitkus Ltd, London.

234

The complete book of
yoga and meditation
for pregnancy

INDEX

236

The complete book of
yoga and meditation
for pregnancy

238

The complete book of
yoga and meditation
for pregnancy

244

The complete book of
yoga and meditation
for pregnancy

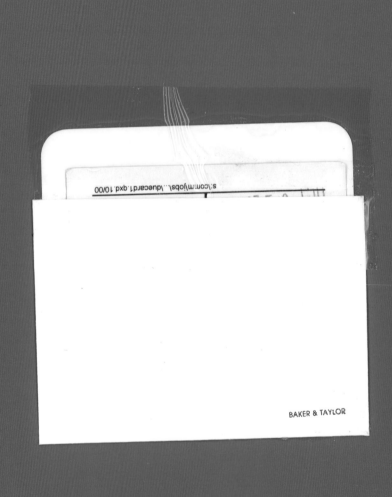